CORONARY ARTERY BYPASS GRAFT SURGERY

Edited by **Wilbert S. Aronow**

Coronary Artery Bypass Graft Surgery
http://dx.doi.org/10.5772/68027
Edited by Wilbert S. Aronow

Contributors
Ragab Hani Donkol, Zizi Saad Mahmoud, Mohammed Elrawy, Marco Gennari, Natalia Bezdenezhnykh, Alexei Sumin, Olga Barbarash, Andrey Bezdenezhnykh, Takashi Murashita, Bandar Al-Ghamdi, Omer Tanyeli, Naomi Kondo Nakagawa, Priscila Aikawa, Felipe Paulitsch, Guillermo Mazzucco, Renata Gomes Paulitsch, Frank Manetta, Allan Mattia

Published by InTech
Janeza Trdine 9, 51000 Rijeka, Croatia

Publishing Process Manager Renata Sliva
Technical Editor SPi Global
Cover InTech Design team

First published December, 2017
Printed in Croatia
Legal deposit, Croatia: National and University Library in Zagreb

Additional hard copies can be obtained from orders@intechopen.com

Coronary Artery Bypass Graft Surgery, Edited by Wilbert S. Aronow
p. cm.
Print ISBN 978-953-51-3709-2
Online ISBN 978-953-51-3710-8

Meet the editor

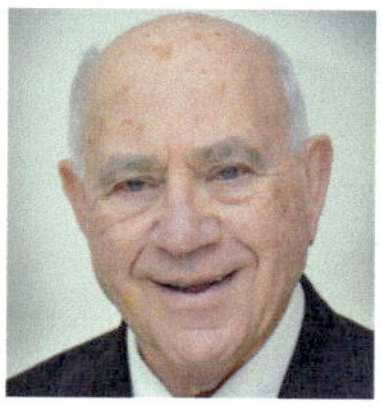

Wilbert S. Aronow MD is Professor of Medicine and Director of Cardiology Research at New York Medical College/Westchester Medical Center, Valhalla, NY, USA. Dr. Aronow received his MD from Harvard Medical School. He has edited 16 books and is author or co-author of 1,605 papers, 441 commentaries, 47 Letters to the Editor, and 1,075 abstracts and is presenter or co-presenter of 1,442 talks at meetings. Dr. Aronow is a Fellow of the ACC, the AHA, the ACP, the ACCP, the ASPC, the AGS (Founding Fellow of Western Section), and the GSA. He has been a member of 162 editorial boards of medical journals, a member of 4 national guidelines committees, and has received numerous teaching and research awards.

Contents

Preface

The book Coronary Artery Bypass Graft Surgery is an excellent update for health care professionals, taking care of patients who are being considered for or who have had coronary artery bypass graft surgery. The 8 chapters in this book are all written by experts in their topics.

The first chapter discusses the role of computed tomography coronary angiography in the evaluation of coronary artery bypass grafts. Graft patency assessment by computed tomography coronary angiography is appropriate in symptomatic patients at risk for graft stenosis/occlusion and has high diagnostic accuracy in assessing graft patency. The use of the left internal mammary artery improves long-term survival and is the gold standard in coronary artery bypass grafting. The choice of second or third graft conduit is controversial. The second chapter discusses the choice of graft conduits in coronary artery bypass grafting. The third chapter discusses current treatment options for significant left main coronary artery disease. Left main coronary disease with low SYNTAX scores (≤22) can be treated with either coronary artery bypass graft surgery or by percutaneous coronary intervention. Patients with a SYNTAX score >32 should only be treated by coronary artery bypass graft surgery. Diabetes mellitus is a major risk factor for coronary artery disease. The fourth chapter discusses the management of diabetes mellitus and other coronary risk factor control in diabetics undergoing coronary revascularization. The fifth chapter discusses the incidence, etiology, pathogenesis, and surgical strategies to prevent neurological complications in patients undergoing coronary artery bypass graft surgery.

Cardiac arrhythmias are common after coronary artery bypass graft surgery and contribute to cardiovascular morbidity and mortality. Chapter 6 discusses the management of cardiac arrhythmias after coronary artery bypass graft surgery. Exercise-based rehabilitation is a very important adjunct treatment for secondary prevention of cardiovascular events and mortality in patients with coronary artery disease and should be used in all patients after coronary artery bypass graft surgery. Chapter 7 discusses physical training programs after coronary artery bypass graft surgery. Coronary artery disease is the most common cause of death in developed countries. Chapter 8 discusses in a very comprehensive manner the medical and surgical management and outcomes for coronary artery disease.

In conclusion, this excellent book provides the practicing physician and other healthcare personnel, who take care of patients with coronary artery disease, new information valuable in his or her care of patients with coronary artery disease.

Wilbert S. Aronow, MD, FACC, FAHA, FCCP, FACP
Professor of Medicine and Director of Cardiology Research,
Westchester Medical Center and New York Medical College,
Valhalla, NY, USA

Section 1

Coronary Artery Bypass Graft Surgery

Chapter 1

Evaluation of Coronary Artery Bypass by CT Coronary Angiography

Ragab Hani Donkol, Zizi Saad Mahmoud and
Mohammed Elrawy

Additional information is available at the end of the chapter

http://dx.doi.org/10.5772/intechopen.70439

Abstract

Coronary computed tomography angiography (CCTA) is an accurate method for graft imaging and assessment than invasive coronary angiography (ICA). CTA has excellent sensitivity and specificity. The chapter describes the role of CTA in evaluation of coronary bypass graft. It covers the appropriate indications for performing CTA after bypass operation, patient preparation, as well as protocol and technique of CTA. The chapter describes the post-examination processing of the images and how to interpret CTA images for detection of graft patency or dysfunction as occlusion, partial thrombosis, poor blood flow, and stealing flow from native artery. According to the American College of Cardiology, the American College of Radiology, and the North American Society for Cardiovascular Imaging, graft patency assessment with CTA is an appropriate approach in symptomatic patients at risk for graft stenosis/occlusion. Cardiac CT can be used to assess the patency of coronary artery bypass graft (CABG) with high diagnostic accuracy compared with ICA and even with a better performance compared to the assessment of native coronaries.

Keywords: CT coronary angiography, coronary artery bypass graft, arterial graft, venous graft, coronary graft failure

1. Introduction

The standard of care for management of advanced coronary artery disease is coronary artery bypass graft (CABG) surgery. The long-term clinical outcome after myocardial revascularization depends on the patency of the coronary artery bypass grafts [1].

Percutaneous coronary angiography is the conventional diagnostic modality to evaluate the coronary arteries and grafts. It is considered the gold standard tool to assess bypass graft status in post-CABG surgery patients. However, invasive coronary angiography (ICA) is invasive, risky, and costly procedure [1].

Advances in technology makes multidetector computed tomography (MDCT) a reliable imaging modality for evaluation of coronary artery bypass graft. The coronary bypass grafts are superior to native coronary arteries for imaging as they are less influenced by cardiac motion, have a wider luminal diameter, and are less calcified. CT coronary angiography (CTA) is a relatively painless noninvasive procedure when compared to invasive coronary angiography, and it is well tolerated by most of the patients. All these causes make CTA a primary method in evaluation graft patency and dysfunction.

2. Evaluation of coronary artery bypass by CT coronary angiography

2.1. Types of coronary bypass grafts

Depending on the approach used for revascularization, the surgeon can utilize different types of arterial and venous grafts. The outcome of coronary artery bypass grafting is closely related to the type of graft either venous or arterial. Arterial grafts are commonly used because of a better patency rate than venous coronary artery bypass grafts [2].

2.1.1. Venous grafts

Venous bypass grafts still represent the majority of all grafts used for bypass surgery. Venous bypass grafts are typically larger in diameter than the native large epicardial coronary arteries (approximately 4–10 mm versus 2–5 mm), and they are less subjected to cardiac motion. Although arterial grafts have better long-term patency rate and outcome, venous grafts, specifically saphenous vein grafts (SVGs), are more readily available. The great saphenous vein (GSV) is usually directly anastomosed to the aorta to revascularize any coronary artery both in a single graft (**Figure 1**) and in a sequential arrangement (**Figure 2**).

There are many causes of venous bypass graft dysfunction. According to the post-operative period, very early after surgery till few weeks after surgery, technical deficiencies and thrombotic activation lead to thrombotic occlusion in approximately 5–10% of the grafts. Then, the two major causes of graft failure within the first year after surgery are intimal hyperplasia and thrombosis, with an occlusion rate of 10–15% [3].

Finally, after the first year, atherosclerosis mechanisms predominate. After 5 years, atherothrombotic occlusion of venous grafts accounts for a reduced patency rate. It has traditionally been estimated to range between 40 and 60% at 10–12 years [2, 4].

2.1.2. Arterial grafts.

As a rule, arterial grafts are smaller in caliber than venous grafts. In the order of frequency of use, graft arteries include the internal mammary arteries (IMAs), radial arteries (RAs), right

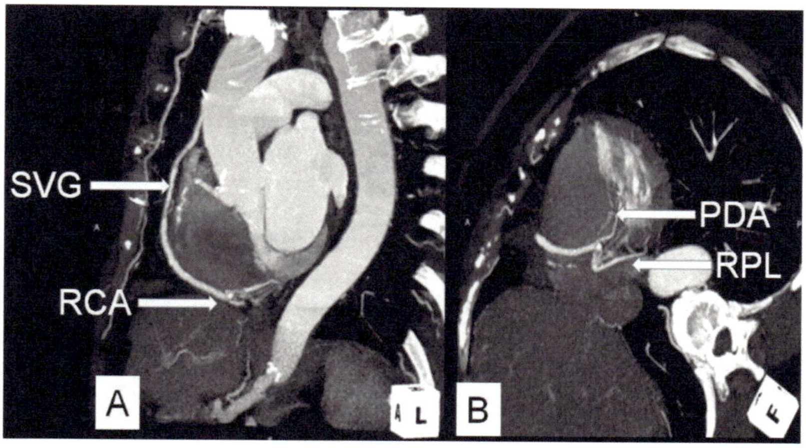

Figure 1. An example of a patent single venous graft in a 63-year-old male patient who underwent saphenous vein graft (SVG) to distal right coronary artery (RCA) with well-opacified distal branches; the posterior descending artery (PDA) and right posterolateral branch (RPL). The figure shows maximum intensity projection images (MIP) of CTA in the sagittal (panel A) and oblique (panel B) planes.

gastroepiploic artery, and inferior epigastric artery. The left internal mammary artery (LIMA) is most often used in coronary bypass arterial grafts. The walls of the arterial graft vessels are much better adapted to the high systemic blood pressure and shear stress mechanism than the

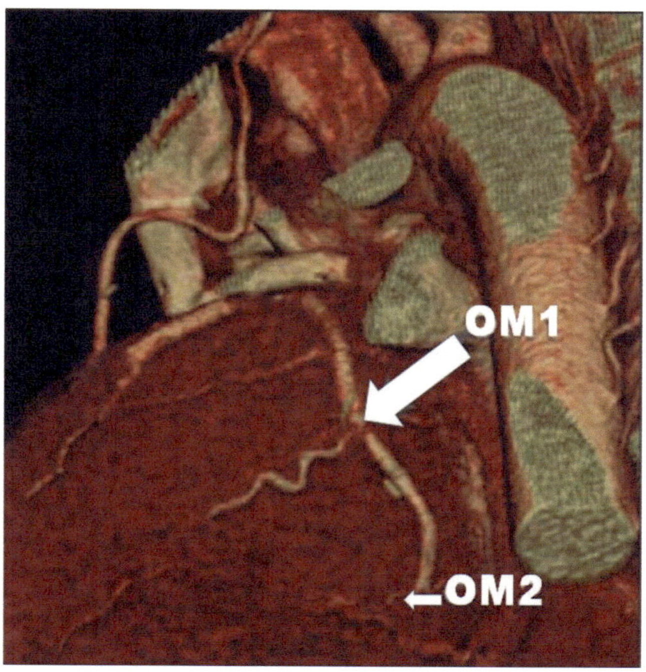

Figure 2. An example of a patent sequential venous graft in a 68-year-old male patient who underwent saphenous vein graft (SVG) to the first and second obtuse marginal arteries (OM1 and OM2). The image is a 3D volume rendering of CTA which was performed because of inconclusive stress test.

walls of the veins, and this leads to improved patency rates of the arterial grafts. If IMA grafts are patent at 1 week after surgery, they will have a 10-year patency rate of 88% [5].

The location and status of the recipient coronary artery influence the graft survival rate. Better survival rate was demonstrated for LIMA bypass grafts and in the situations where the diameter of the native coronary artery is ≥2 mm. However, internal mammary grafts to a recipient vessel with <50% diameter stenosis may have a very high rate of occlusion, probably due to competing flow through the native vessel [5].

Arterial grafts pose some limitations to CTA study, as is the presence of metallic clips in mammary artery and, particularly, in radial artery grafts, which interfere with the visualization of lesions. Also, the nondynamic nature of CTA makes the assessment of competitive flow or vasospasm in the arterial graft difficult [2, 4, 6].

The arterial grafts are usually anastomosed as follows [7]:

- The left internal mammary artery is usually anastomosed to the left descending coronary artery, diagonals, and/or obtuse marginal branches both in a single graft (**Figure 3**) and in a sequential arrangement.
- The right internal mammary artery (RIMA) is usually anastomosed to the left anterior descending coronary artery crossing the midline (**Figure 4**), to the proximal right coronary artery, to obtuse marginal branches or diagonals, via the transverse sinus (behind the aorta), or to obtuse branches or diagonals.
- The radial artery is also used as free graft to all coronary arteries as a single graft or in sequential arrangement. It is more frequently attached in a Y-configuration to left or right internal mammary grafts and less commonly to the ascending aorta.
- The gastroepiploic artery is only rarely used to revascularize the posterior descending coronary artery; sometimes, it is used as a free graft to extend a left internal mammary graft anastomosed to the very distal part of left anterior descending coronary artery.

2.1.3. Planning for grafting

During CABG surgery, if multiple grafts are planned, during surgery they arranged from above downward to avoid crossover of the grafts. Grafts arising from the right side of the ascending aorta are arranged to the right coronary superiorly and posterior descending artery inferiorly. While on the left side, grafts are arranged to circumflex, obtuse marginal, diagonal, and left descending arteries from above downward, respectively.

2.2. Coronary CT angiography technical requirements and protocol

2.2.1. CT scanner

The advancement in the technology of computed tomography (CT) makes CT coronary angiography a popular diagnostic modality for evaluation of coronary arteries and bypass grafts.

http://dx.doi.org/10.5772/intechopen.70439

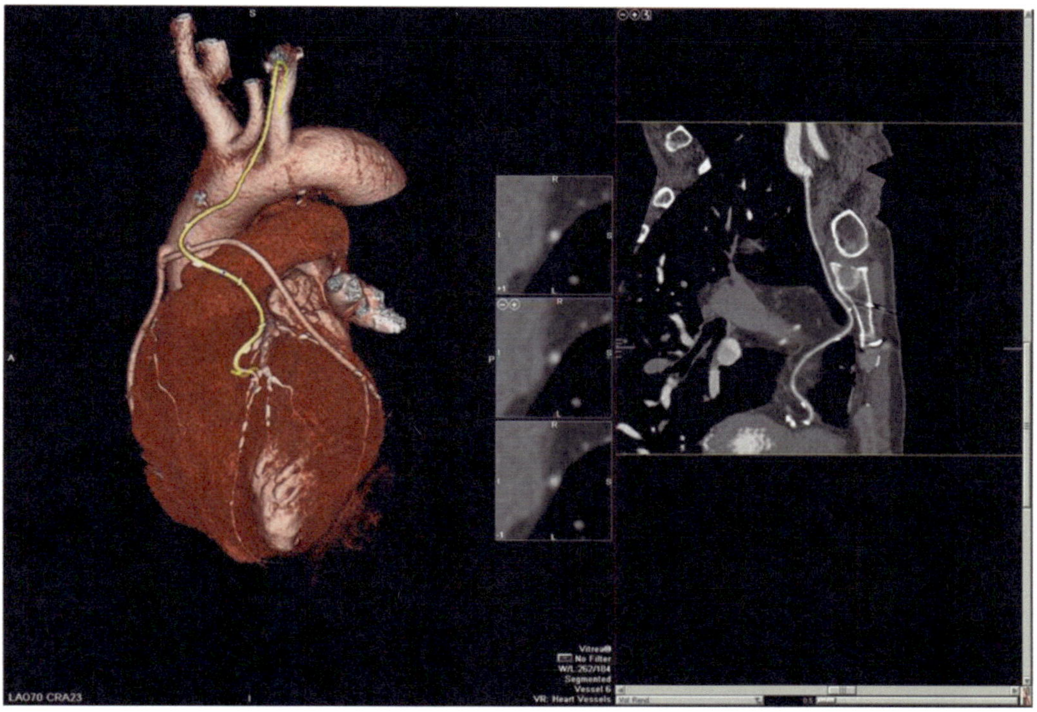

Figure 3. A patent left internal mammary artery (LIMA) graft anastomosed to the left anterior descending (LAD) coronary artery in a 62-year-old male patient who has inconclusive stress echo test.

CT is a noninvasive procedure and well tolerated by many patients. The recent multislice or multidetector CT (MDCT) has a faster gantry rotation with high temporal and spatial resolutions. Also, MDCT has a high X-ray tube potential and wide field of scan. Therefore, MDCT gives a short scanning time, better image quality, and lower patient radiation dose. CT of coronary artery bypass grafts requires a larger scan range (12.5–22.0 cm) and consequently a longer breath hold. Sixty-four-row MDCT scanners or more make CTA of coronary artery bypasses a practical approach with a short breath-hold duration (12–15 s) and thin-slice imaging. Nowadays, for clinical routine, at least 64-row scanners are recommended for follow-up of patients after coronary bypass surgery.

2.2.2. *Patient preparation*

For patients with high or irregular heart rate, beta-adrenergic blockers are given prior to CT scan to prevent motion artifacts secondary to heart rate variability and tachycardia. It is better to scan patient with low heart rate ranging from 60 to 70 beats per minute. To avoid respiratory motion artifacts, patients are scanned with breath-holding (mid-inspiration period). It is better to scan patients while fasting for about 6 h before the study without dehydration. The patients must have normal renal function and are free of adverse contrast media reaction during any past radiological studies.

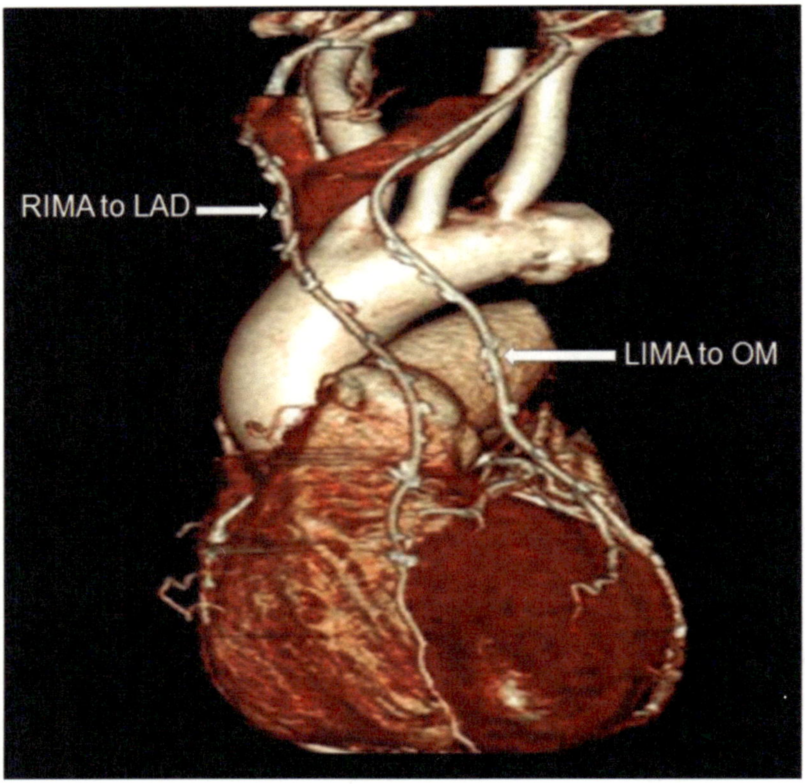

Figure 4. Three-dimensional reconstructions of CAA in a 65-year-old male patient who underwent right internal mammary artery (RIMA) to the left anterior descending (LAD) coronary artery and left internal mammary artery (LIMA) grafting to an obtuse marginal (OM) branch. Both grafts are patent.

2.2.3. MDCT acquisition protocols

There are a variety of protocols for image acquisition in the evaluation of patients after CABG surgery. In many respects, the protocols are similar to that for coronary CT angiography.

If the heart rate are slow and stable (less than 70 beats per minute), it is recommended to use the protocol of sequential prospective ECG triggering with padding. This protocol has the advances of reduction of the patient's total radiation dose by about 80–90% compared to retrospective scanning protocol. The drawbacks of prospective ECG-triggering acquisition are a lack of flexibility in reconstructing image data across the cardiac cycle and the impossibility to undertake functional analysis unless single-beat prospective triggering with tube current modulation is used.

On the other hand, patients with previous bypass graft surgery often have irregular and high heart rates. So, in those patients we use the retrospective spiral ECG-gating protocol which has the advantage of potential flexibility in reconstructing image data at different cardiac cycles to choose the best phase with the least cardiac motion. Also, retrospective protocol has the advantage of performing cardiac functional analysis.

2.2.4. *Technical parameters of the scan*

The scan range depends on both the modalities of grafting. For patients who have received an internal mammary artery bypass graft, the scan should be extended superiorly to include the origins of the internal mammary arteries from the subclavian arteries (at the middle of the clavicle). The scan usually ends at the inferior border of the heart with the exception of patients with a gastroepiploic artery graft, in whom the scan has to include the upper abdomen.

During scanning, patients are placed in the CT table in the supine feet-first position. The duration of the scan ranges from 10 to 15 s. The images are acquired in a limited field of view with axial images centered on the heart. Scanning is performed in a caudal-to-cranial direction to obtain images of the main bulk of the heart and coronary arteries during the initial phase of the acquisition when breath-holding is most effective. The tube potential is 100–120 kVp according to the patient built with tube current of 800 mAs and pitch of 0.2.

2.2.5. *Contrast media*

Cardiac CTA technique requires rapid injection of nonionic, iodinated, low osmolar intravenous contrast media. Right-sided injection of contrast is preferred to avoid venous contrast crossing grafts. An amount of approximately 60–100 ml of contrast agent followed by a saline flush is sufficient for bypass imaging using 64-MDCT using a dual-head injector.

To optimize the opacification of the coronary arteries, and bypass grafts, an anatomic, automatic triggering method either bolus-tracking or timing bolus technique is used with 8–10 s delay after injection. In the bolus-tracking technique, a threshold of 150 HU is preset at the region of interest (ROI) in the descending aorta. In the timing bolus technique, the ROI in the ascending aorta and scanning will be started immediately at the time of maximum density of the curve. Bolus tracking is preferred for more consistent results and more homogeneous contrast in the coronary arteries.

2.2.6. *Post-processing reconstruction*

An advanced diagnostic workstation is required for post-processing reconstruction of the axial source images. Three-dimensional volume rendering (3DVRT) is particularly useful in patients who underwent surgical revascularization because it allows a quick overview of arterial and venous grafts and a quick evaluation of their anatomical condition. This should be supplemented by oblique multiplanar reformations (MPR) and curved multiplanar reformations (cMPR) which allows quantification of percent diameter stenosis on cross sections along the vessel. Significant stenoses are usually searched for by scrolling through axial images with and without maximum intensity projection (MIP).

Analysis capabilities of the machine are required in cases examined by retrospective ECG gating for assigning the cardiac anatomy and functions as well as valvular and wall motion abnormalities. Sharp kernels are used for stent imaging and in heavily calcified vessels, which are common in patients after bypass grafting.

2.3. The value of CTA in the context of cardiovascular imaging for CABG assessment

Echocardiography and MRI have recognized weaknesses in terms direct visualization of the coronary arteries or bypass grafts. CT coronary angiography is more sensitive and specific than echocardiography and MRI in imaging of coronary arteries and bypass grafts [4].

Conventional coronary angiography has so far been considered the reference standard for visualization of both native coronary arteries and bypass grafts. Evaluation by ICA in patients with prior CABG can be challenging and exposes patients to large contrast volumes in addition to rare complications such as injury to the graft vessel during catheter engagement.

With its inherent advantages and good diagnostic accuracy, noninvasive coronary angiography using CT is considered a viable alternative in symptomatic patients after coronary artery bypass grafting. Coronary artery bypass grafts are more amenable to CTA imaging, due to their larger diameter and lower pulsatile movements along the cardiac cycle than native arteries and their relative freedom from calcification. CT was first proposed for noninvasive imaging of coronary artery venous bypass grafts by Brundage et al. in 1980 [8]. However, at that time the detection of flow-limiting stenoses was not possible. Improved CT technology has since greatly improved, which has important implications for the diagnostic evaluation of bypass grafts. A relevant aspect of MDCT study of CABG is its ability to readily define the status of patency or occlusion of the graft, being in this sense equal or even superior to invasive angiography. However, applicability of CT to all patients is limited by premature atrial or ventricular contractions, which can reduce image quality when occurring during scanning. Moreover, in patients with coronary artery bypass grafts, the investigation of the native vessels can pose a challenge because of the severe coronary calcifications present.

CT coronary angiography has a very important role for CABG assessment and to avoid invasive coronary angiography. This role is termed as the potential "gatekeeper" role of CTA in the meta-analysis study performed by Barbero et al. They concluded that ICA has a higher cost compared to CTA, and it is inconvenient for most of the patients due to the need for sedation with resultant driving restrictions, as well as a low risk of stroke, infarction, dissection, arrhythmia, or death. On the other hand, CTA is a noninvasive procedure, and it is highly accepted by patients [9].

2.4. Accuracy of different generations of CT in coronary bypass graft assessment

Initial investigation of bypass grafts was done with single-slice scanners, and electron beam CT in1997 by Achenbach et al., who evaluated hemodynamically relevant stenosis, was possible in 84% of the cases with some limitation in the scan due to breathing artifacts and misplacement of the imaging volume [2].

Subsequently, the addition of electrocardiographic (ECG) gating and the improved capabilities available with 4- or 16-slice MDCT scanners for rapid scanning of the area of interest led to promising results in the imaging of bypass grafts.

Four-row CT provided an anisotropic resolution, which oftentimes did not depict the distal anastomosis, and 38% of the patent grafts could not be evaluated because of respiratory/

motion/metallic clip artifacts [10, 11]. Sixteen-row CT scanners improved assessment of occlusion/significant stenosis; however, about 20% were not assessable because of artifacts [12, 13].

The introduction of 64-slice MDCT and dual-source CT permitted improved temporal resolution (up to 83 ms), spatial resolution ($0.4 \times 0.4 \times 0.4\ mm^3$), and reduction of both cardiac and respiratory motion, leading to improved assessment of arterial and venous graft stenosis and occlusion. Reports on diagnostic accuracy of MDCT in CABG have shown values of sensitivity and specificity over 95% for the presence of lesions in these vessels. However, the investigation of native vessels showed that sensitivity and specificity are significantly lower than in patients with suspected coronary artery disease [14–18].

In the meta-analysis study performed by Dr. Barbero and colleagues, they reviewed 10 different studies of 959 patients post coronary bypass operations with 1586 arterial and venous grafts. These patents were evaluated using 64-multidector CT scanners of different vendors. The overall sensitivity and specificity of CT coronary angiography in detecting complete graft occlusions were 99 and 99%, respectively, as compared to invasive coronary angiography. They also performed meta-analysis of 12 different studies of 2482 bypass grafts and found that the sensitivity and specificity of CTA in detecting significant graft stenosis (with more than 50% diameter reduction) was 98% regardless the age of patients or the post-operative period after CABG surgery [13].

The introduction of 128-, 256-, and 320-multislice CT gave high temporal and spatial resolution with a less cardiac and respiratory motion, improving assessment of bypass graft patency, stenosis, or occlusion with a promising results. This improvement in image quality allows a comprehensive assessment of the grafts and the native vessels [19–21].

2.5. The appropriate indications of CTCA in CABG assessment

One of the appropriate indications of CTA is imaging and follow-up of symptomatic patients with coronary artery bypass grafts (e.g., recurrent chest pain). In cases of suspected graft failure, post-CABG recurrent symptoms may be due to disease progression, commonly in native coronary arteries, in the venous grafts, or less commonly in an arterial grafts.

There are specific clinical conditions which may favor the use of CT angiography over invasive coronary angiography for graft evaluation as in patients with a positive cardiac test suggesting possible ischemic disease in the territory of a specific coronary bypass graft when disease distal to the graft anastomosis seems less likely. Also, CT coronary angiography is helpful in some patients where an anatomic correlation may be required following an equivocal functional cardiac test. Another clinical situation in evaluation of cases showed borderline graft stenosis or change in symptoms. CTA may be helpful in assessment of patients when the proximal grafts may be affected by other vascular diseases as vasculitis or formation of true or false aneurysms of the bypass graft [22].

Another appropriate indication is to know the course of previously grafted IMA prior to redo-CABG. CTA evaluates patients with unknown previous CABG surgical details to know the number, location, and pathways of grafts before planning management by invasive coronary angiography. CT coronary angiography before invasive coronary angiography has the potential to the procedure faster and more efficient due to an improved understanding of topography of graft anatomy before attempting to engage graft ostia and evaluate graft body and distal coronary perfusion by percutaneous coronary catheter. However, the combined approach to evaluate CABG by both CTA and ICA results in a higher radiation and contrast dose [22, 23].

2.6. The limitations of CTCA in CABG assessment

Patients with significant obesity (e.g., body mass index >40 kg/m^2) or who have irregular heart rhythms may not be ideal candidates for CTA. In addition those with stage 4 chronic kidney disease (CKD) with glomerular filtration rate below 30 mL/min are also not good candidates for CTA. CTA has limitation in scanning individuals with a large number of metallic surgical clips as clips may interfere in assessment degree of stenosis of the graft itself and the distal anastomosis [4, 24].

2.7. Systematic approach for graft assessment

Before starting CT image interpretation, the surgical report and last cardiac catheter report showed be reviewed. Then, the images are preferred to be read according to the following systemic sequences for complete and accurate image interpretation:

- Check the axial, sagittal, and coronal views of the chest wall to know if RIMA and LIMA are present or not, also the status of the surgical wires (intact or ruptured) and the sternum for dehiscence and infection (**Figure 5**).
- Volume-rendered images: for a rapid overview of graft anatomy to identify the type and course of the venous and arterial grafts as well as the presence of stumps and pledgets (**Figure 6**).
- Comprehensive graft evaluation by scrolling the axial images and MPR images to assess patency of the bypass grafts and run-off, proximal, and distal graft anastomoses. In particular, curved planar images (cMPR) with centerlines through the bypass grafts using rotation tool to attempt elimination of clip effect (**Figure 7**).
- If possible assess the native coronary arteries.
- Examine anatomy of the thoracic aorta and left ventricle (diastolic dimensions).
- If the study is retrospective spiral CT, assess left ventricular and valve functions.

2.8. Imaging findings and interpretation

2.8.1. Bypass graft patency

Interpretation of CTA following CABG surgery is started first by assessing the morphology and size of the ascending aorta and the origin of the in situ vessel (in the case of an in situ vessel, such as the IMA). Then, graft patency is assessed along its whole length. Diagnosis of graft patency can be diagnosed if there is uniform homogeneous enhancement of the graft lumen by injecting contrast with smooth outline of the wall of the graft wall. For systematic

http://dx.doi.org/10.5772/intechopen.70439

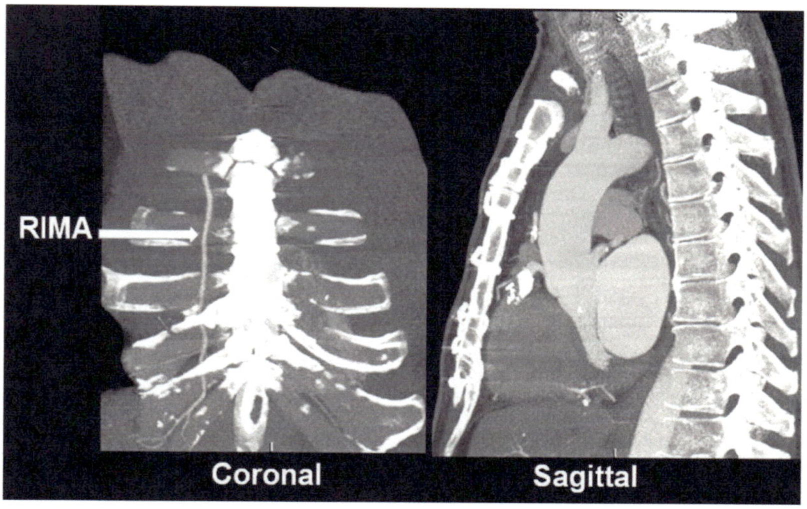

Figure 5. Coronal and sagittal reconstructed images of CTA of post-CABG surgery showing the status of the chest wall. The images show good healed sternum with intact wires. The left internal mammary artery (LIMA) is not in its normal position (repositioned for arterial graft), while the right internal mammary artery (RIMA) is present in its place.

evaluation of the graft, it is divided into three different segments: the origin or proximal anastomosis, the body, and the distal anastomosis of the graft. Usually, the proximal anastomosis of the graft is accurately assessed than the distal anastomosis due to its better visualization by CTA. In some cases where the distal anastomosis is not well visualized, the bypass graft is considered patent if there is homogeneous contrast enhancement of its lumen.

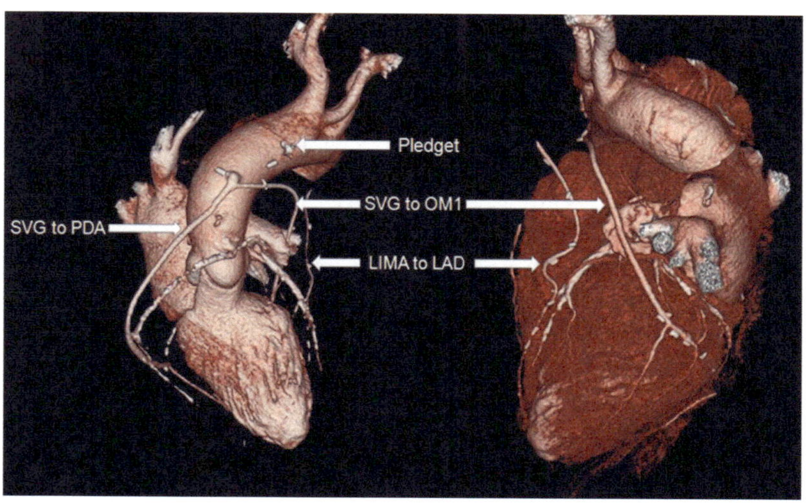

Figure 6. Volume-rendering reconstructed images of CTA of post-CABG showing the type and course of multiple different bypass grafts. The images show grafted saphenous vein graft (SVG) to posterior descending artery (PDA), left internal mammary artery (LIMA) to left anterior descending artery (LAD), and SVG to first obtuse marginal (OM1) artery. The three grafts are patent, and the native coronary arteries show different grades of stenosis. A high-attenuation felt pledget is depicted at the distal portion of the ascending aorta. Note that the high-attenuation focus is located external to the aortic wall.

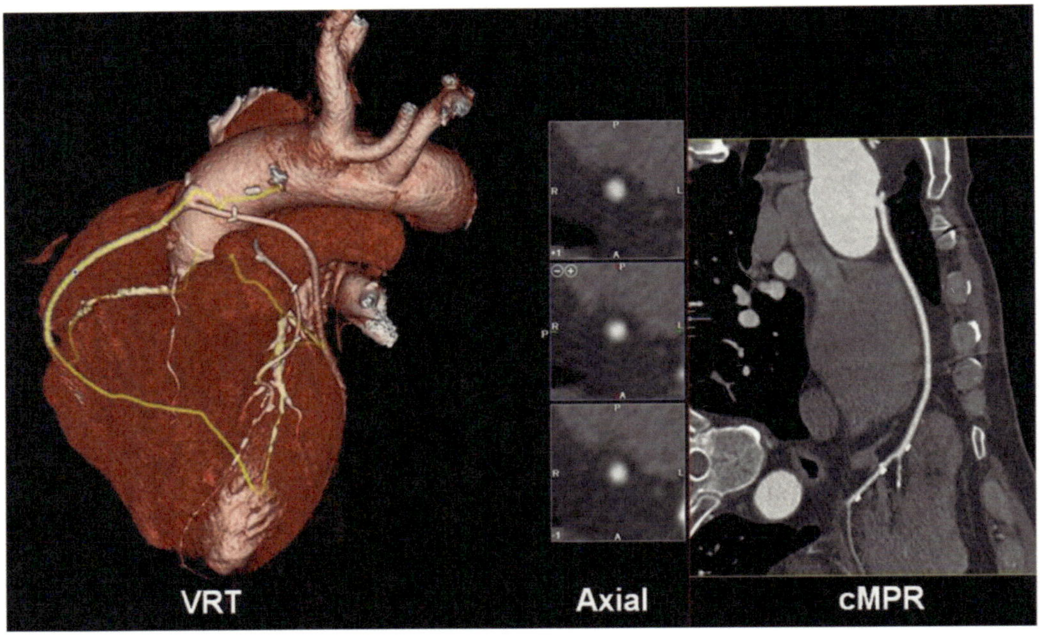

Figure 7. The comprehensive approach to track a saphenous vein graft to the posterior descending artery in 3D virtual reconstruction (VRT) and axial and curved multiplanar reconstruction images (cMPR). The tracking line in the VRT images delineates the graft from its origin to the distal anastomosis. Axial images show the cross section of the graft lumen to determine the degree of diameter reduction and status of the wall. cMPR images are rotating through the bypass graft to eliminate the blooming effect of clips. Note that the graft is patent with a normal distal anastomosis.

Outcome of the graft patency differs according to its type and anastomosis. General patency of IMA grafts was better than for SVGs, and patency of SVG graft in LAD or D1 was better than its placement in PDA or OM artery. The patency of the grafts and presence of significant stenosis (>50% reduction in graft diameter at any point along its length by visual estimation) were evaluated. Recognize artifacts associated with surgical clips as blooming and beam hardening. The nonrevascularized native coronary arteries and those with incomplete revascularization were assessed by segments, following the 17-segment American College of Cardiology/American Heart Association (ACC/AHA) model 17 [25].

2.8.2. Bypass graft failure

Recognizing the appearances of graft complications is an essential part of the radiologist's interpretation of post-bypass CTA imaging.

2.8.2.1. Stenosis and occlusion of the graft

Failures of the graft can occur early or late after CABG surgery.

Early graft failure usually occurs within 1 month after surgery, and its main reason is vessel thrombosis from platelet dysfunction at the site of focal damage of the lining endothelium during surgical intervention. There are other factors that also initiate early venous graft failure such as the hypercoagulability state of the patient and the high-pressure distension or stretching of the venous graft, with its intrinsically weaker antithrombotic features. These factors contribute for 3–12% occlusion rate within the first post-operative month [26].

The cause of delayed venous graft failure is due to progressive physiopathological changes related to the exposure of their wall to the systemic blood pressure which results in neointimal hyperplasia. By itself neointimal hyperplasia does not produce luminal occlusion or stenosis. But later on it will be the seat for development of atheroma and thrombosis of the venous graft. One year after surgery, the main cause of graft failure is atherosclerosis. The arterial grafts, specifically IMA grafts, are more resistant to formation of atheroma than the venous grafts. However, the main reason for late IMA graft failure is progression of atherosclerotic disease in the native coronary artery distal to the graft anastomosis [26].

Univariate analysis was performed in the study of Esam et al. in 2016 to find out the probable risk factors for graft occlusion such as age (>65 years), post-CABG duration >5 years, hypertension, diabetes, dyslipidemia, smoking, diffuse CAD, and LV dysfunction. Surprisingly, the statistical analysis could not demonstrate any cardiac risk factors which could significantly be associated with graft patency or occlusion [27].

The imaging findings associated with graft stenosis and occlusion can be easily diagnosed by CTA as the presence of calcified, mixed, and noncalcified atherosclerotic plaques. The estimation of the extent and degree of diameter reduction can be easily performed by post-processing images of CTA. Graft occlusion can be easily diagnosed by nonvisualization of the lumen of the graft after revision of the previous grafting surgical report (**Figure 8**).

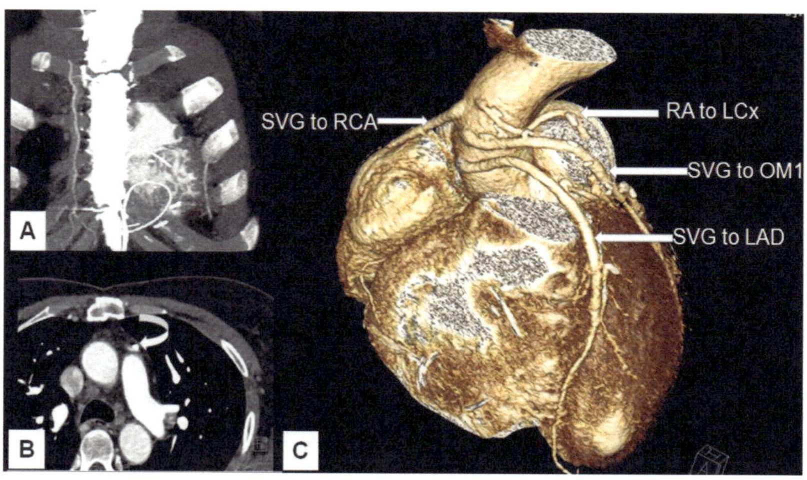

Figure 8. A 72-year-old male patient who was operated 10 years earlier with four grafts: left internal mammary artery graft to left anterior descending artery (LIMA to LAD), saphenous vein graft to right coronary artery (SVG to RCA), radial graft to left circumflex artery (RA to LCx), and SVG to first obtuse marginal (SVG to OM1). Because of an occlusion of LIMA to LAD graft and typical chest pain, redo-bypass graft surgery was performed 4 years ago with SVG to LAD to revascularize LAD. Post second operation CTA was performed because of atypical chest pain. Carnal (panel A) and axial (panel B) images showed absent LIMA with occlusion of the old LIMA to LAD graft (curved arrow). VRT image (panel C) showed patent all old and new venous grafts, but the arterial graft (RA to LCx) is occluded midway between its origin and distal anastomosis.

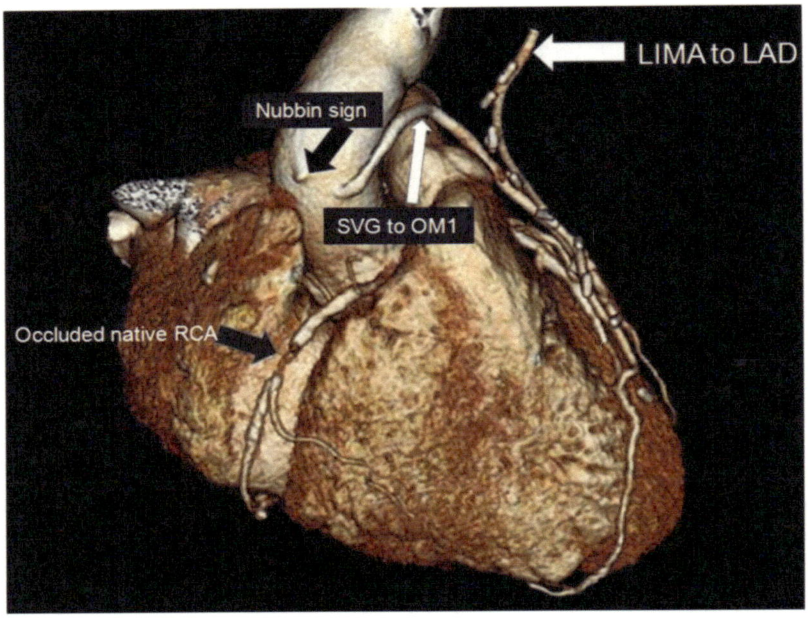

Figure 9. A 65-year-old male patient who underwent left internal mammary artery to left anterior descending artery graft (LIMA to LAD) as well as two venous grafts, saphenous vein graft to right coronary artery (SVG to RCA), and SVG to first obtuse marginal branch (SVG to OM1) 7 years ago. CTA was performed because of recurrence of atypical angina. Volume-rendering images showed that the LIMA to LAD and SVG to OM1 grafts are patent. The image showed the nubbin sign along the right anterolateral ascending aorta, indicating an occluded SVG to RCA. Additionally, occlusion of the native RCA is seen as well.

In many cases of proximal graft occlusion, the most proximal part of an occluded aortocoronary graft fills with contrast, creating a small contrast-filled outpouching from the ascending aorta known as nubbin sign (**Figure 9**). In some cases a "ghost" of the occluded part of the graft may be visible [1].

In some cases, a felt pledget can be seen in the aorta prior to cannulation sites. The holes are closed with stitching or suturing, which may then be reinforced with prosthetic material such as polytetrafluoroethylene (PTFE) sutures to reinforce suture sites and reduce the tearing of vessels. This hemostatic technique is most often used in elderly patients (>80 years old), who have fragile tissue. The use of felt pledgets increases susceptibility to local bacterial seeding. At CT, felt pledgets are depicted as high-attenuation material (**Figure 7**). It is important to distinguish this nonsignificant post-operative finding from the appearance of other significant findings as a calcified atherosclerotic plaque, a contrast leak, a calcified mediastinal lymph node, or pericardial calcification. The atherosclerotic plaques can be differentiated from the felt pledgets as the later are located on the extraluminal surface of the aorta. Differentiating between a felt pledget and a focal contrast leak can be difficult on the post-contrast CT because the CT attenuation of a felt pledget measured in Hounsfield units can be similar to that of contrast-enhanced blood. This difficulty can be resolved with examination of the nonenhanced CT images, on which the felt pledget remains hyperdense [28].

Acute or chronic graft occlusion can sometimes be differentiated by the diameter of the bypass graft. In chronic occlusion, the diameter is usually reduced from scarring, as compared with acute occlusion in which the diameter is usually enlarged. If graft occluded, carefully examine proximal vessel for severe disease or competitive flow.

2.8.2.2. *Evaluation of native coronary arteries*

In patients who underwent coronary artery bypass grafting, recurrence of symptoms can be due to graft failure or progression of atherosclerosis in the native vessels. While CTA offers excellent accuracy for the detection of bypass graft stenosis or graft occlusion, this test is more limited for evaluating native coronary arteries. The native coronary arteries in patients after bypass grafting are not as easily assessed as are the bypasses themselves, and only a few studies have addressed the combined reading of coronaries and bypasses. The native arteries are very difficult to assess by CT as they often have severe atherosclerosis, including pronounced calcification, and frequently are of small caliber, which makes their evaluation challenging. So if the clinical situation requires assessment of the native coronary artery system only, the value of CTA is limited. However, recent scanner with 128 and 256 MDCT has higher temporal and spatial resolution and may thus allow more reliable assessment of the native coronary system in patients with bypass grafts. There are few studies reporting accuracy of CTA to diagnose stenosis in native ungrafted coronary arteries. Using a 64-MDCT, the reported sensitivity and specificity of CTA in diagnosis of native coronaries were 86–97% and 76–92%, respectively. Despite these results, functional imaging is more practical than CTA in evaluation of the status of the native coronary arteries in patients after coronary bypass surgeries [29].

2.8.2.3. *Graft malposition*

Malposition of the bypass graft is one of the rare causes of early graft failure. If the graft is too long, it may twist or kink. If the graft is too short, it may stretch, a particular problem in severe chronic obstructive lung disease patients. Also, the aortic connector can also play a role in kinking the bypass graft if the vessel is not supported adequately.

2.8.2.4. *Vasospasm of the radial artery graft*

One of the very early post-operative radial artery bypass graft failures is vasospasm of the grafted radial artery. The appearance is similar to severe graft stenosis, although the length of the narrow segment is much longer. This can be avoided by the administration of intraoperative alpha-adrenergic blocking agents or post-operative calcium channel blockers which can overcome many cases of graft vasospasm postoperatively. Arterial spasm is not a late complication for graft failure as the patency rate for radial artery grafts is approximately 92% at 10 years, similar to IMA grafts [30].

2.8.2.5. *Formation of bypass graft aneurysm*

One of the rare complications that can occur after bypass graft surgery is the formation of pseudo or true graft aneurysm.

In the early post-operative period, pseudoaneurysm may be occurred at the anastomosis secondary to infection or tension at these sites, resulting in suture rupture. Late-onset graft aneurysms can be either true or pseudoaneurysms. They are found 5–7 years after surgery and are related to atherosclerotic changes. Graft aneurysms can lead to various complications, including compression on adjacent structures, thrombosis of their lumens, distal embolization of the bypass graft, or the coronaries leading to an acute coronary event and formation of the right atrium or ventricle. One of the risky complications is rupture of the aneurysm leading to massive hemothorax, hemopericardium, or sudden death. Management of graft aneurysm is by surgery however there is no a clear guideline for the critical size of the graft aneurysm before surgical intervention, but a size more than 2 cm has been a cause for concern [4].

2.8.2.6. Formation of pericardial and pleural effusions

Pericardial effusion is a common post-operative complication and can be occurred in about 75% of the patients after CABG surgery. Risk factors for formation of pericardial effusions are post-operative coagulopathy or the use of anticoagulation agents. Pericardial effusions are early complications and occur between 5 and 10 days postoperatively. Most of pericardial effusions are mild and resolve within a month. But in 0.3% of the patients may develop massive pericardial effusion which progresses to cardiac tamponade. Post-CABG surgery pleural effusions are even more common than pericardial effusion and occurred in 89% of the patients in the first week after surgery. These pleural effusions are usually unilateral, mainly left-sided, small in amount, and with no clinical significance [4].

2.8.2.7. Sternal dehiscence and infection

Disruption and infection of median sternotomy wounds are grave complications. It occurs in 0.3–5% of the cases. This problem is associated with a high mortality rate between 14 and 47%.

Diagnosis of sterna dehiscence is usually made clinically; imaging plays an important role to confirm diagnosis. A midline vertical lucency over the sternum of greater than 3 mm is usually abnormal and should raise the suspicion for dehiscence. X-ray examination of the sternum can demonstrate ruptured wires and sternal dehiscence, wire malposition, fracture, and pseudoarthrosis. Displacement of sternal wires can be seen in about 85% of the cases of dehiscence. CT can diagnose normally united sternum by the presence of new bone formation at the sternotomy site without definite bone remodeling in both the anterior and posterior plates. On the other hand, complete sterna nonunion can appear as definite visible sternal separation of both the anterior and posterior plates of the sternum, while incomplete sterna fusion was defined as fusion of one plate and separation of the other.

Risk factors for post-coronary artery bypass graft infection include diabetes mellitus, obesity, complexity of surgery, length of surgical time, and blood transfusion. Three different compartments may be affected by sterna infection: the presternal (cellulitis, sinus tracts, abscess), sternal (osteomyelitis, dehiscence), and retrosternal (mediastinitis, hematoma, abscess). MDCT allows multiplanar reconstruction and windowing, contributing particularly to the evaluation of the sternum. The sagittal plane is useful for determining the disease extent. Sternal wire abnormalities precede clinical detection of dehiscence by a mean of 3 days in 70% of the cases.

CT scan delineates changes in bone configuration, distinguishes insignificant from major infection, and accurately depicts extent of infection. If there is any persistent or recurrent collection, CT-guided needle aspiration can help determine whether a fluid collection is infected or not.

Post-contrast CT scan is important in diagnosis of the extension of infection and help in guidance of treatment. The detection of clear fat planes of the mediastinal structures in CT scan excludes the presence of infection. Mediastinitis can be diagnosed by the presence of diffuse soft tissue infiltrations with or without gas loculi, obliteration of mediastinal fat planes, and formation of hypodense fluid collections. CT is a useful prognostic tool as it can be used for follow-up of patients after medical and surgical management. CT can also help in guidance of percutaneous drainage of intrathoracic abscess or significant fluid collections [31].

2.8.2.8. *Noncardiac complications and incidental findings*

Although the intent of CTA after CABG surgery is to assess bypass graft patency and surgical complications, incidental findings are also frequently detected. 13.1% of the patients in the immediate post-operative period had unsuspected noncardiac findings, including pulmonary embolism, pulmonary nodules, pneumonia, mucous plugging, and pneumothorax. Therefore, radiologists need to be aware of clinically significant findings with possible life-threatening consequences [32].

2.9. Future researches

CT coronary angiography has high sensitivity and specificity for diagnosis of significant stenosis or occlusion of coronary bypass grafts. However, the functional and clinical significance of these lesions needs further cardiac tests. Further studies are needed to determine which CABG patient may be a suitable candidate for CTA to get the best benefits of coronary revascularization. These functional information could be derived in the future from CTA using mathematically modeled Fractional Flow Reserve CT (FFRCT) which still has not undergone validation among patients after CABG surgery. The current limitations of this technology are the cost nonavailability in most cardiac imaging centers and complexity of the post-processing modeling techniques of coronary physiology to get FFRCT. The added value of FFRCT can make CTA a stand-alone test for evaluation of post-CABG patients and to avoid unnecessary invasive diagnostic tests.

Future studies are also needed to address the cost-effectiveness of different cardiac diagnostic tests and resulting coronary intervention to improve post-operative chest pain and reduce future risk of myocardial infarction and death.

It will take long-term follow-up studies with CTA versus invasive angiography to demonstrate net cost savings in terms of total healthcare expenditures and quality of life years saved as a result of making such interventions.

Future researches may also be needed to explore the potential use of CTA to screen patients for early graft failure immediately following CABG or at different time intervals as identifying candidates for intervention earlier may improve longer-term outcomes. This would require further investigation via a prospective trial that would need to assess patient outcomes in addition to downstream costs and resource utilization.

Subclinical occlusion of the bypass graft may exist for years, because of competitive antegrade or collateral flow; however, CTA does not have the ability to determine the hemodynamic significance of such lesions, which may be unpredictable in the presence of collateral perfusion of the myocardium. So, the assessment of the significance of subclinical occlusion of the graft may require some kind of stress myocardial perfusion by CTA alone or combined with other stress tests.

2.10. Conclusions

CT angiography has a high accuracy for the detection of bypass graft stenosis and occlusion. In recent years, advanced technology of CTA allows cardiovascular imaging physician to evaluate bypass graft patency and malfunction noninvasively with greater confidence. In addition, bypass grafts themselves have a larger caliber than native coronary arteries, and they are subjected to less motion artifacts which favorably influences image quality. Post-contrast CT can also help in diagnosis of other noncoronary complications that may cause post-operative chest pain. Thus, it is very important that every cardiovascular imaging radiologist or cardiologist must be familiar with the different types of coronary bypass grafts, possible early and late post-operative complications, and other incidental imaging findings to maximize the effectiveness of CTA in evaluation of patients after CABG surgery.

Author details

Ragab Hani Donkol[1]*, Zizi Saad Mahmoud[2] and Mohammed Elrawy[2]

*Address all correspondence to: ragabhani@hotmail.com

1 Radiology Department, Faculty of Medicine, Cairo University, Cairo, Egypt

2 Cardiology Department, Zagazig University, Zagazig, Egypt

References

[1] Harskamp RE, Alexander JH, Ferguson TB Jr, Hager R, Mack MJ, Englum B, et al. Frequency and predictors of internal mammary artery graft failure and subsequent clinical outcomes: Insights from the PREVENT IV trial. Circulation. 2016;**133**(2):131-138 https://doi.org/10.1161/CIRCULATIONAHA.115.015549

[2] Achenbach S, Moshage W, Ropers D, et al. Noninvasive, three-dimensional visualization of coronary artery bypass grafts by electron beam tomography. The American Journal of Cardiology. 1997;**79**:856-861 https://doi.org/10.1016/S0002-9149(97)00003-9

[3] Lytle BW, Loop FD, Cosgrove DM, Ratliff NB, Easley K, Taylor PC. Long-term (5 to 12 years) serial studies of internal mammary artery and saphenous vein coronary bypass grafts. The Journal of Thoracic and Cardiovascular Surgery. 1985;**89**:248-258

[4] Dewey M. Cardiac CT. 2nd ed. Berlin Heidelberg: Springer; 2014 https://doi.org/10.1007/978-3-642-41883-9

[5] Owens CD. Adaptive changes in autogenous vein grafts for arterial reconstruction: Clinical implications. Journal of Vascular Surgery. 2010;**51**:736-746 https://doi.org/10.1016/j.jvs.2009.07.102

[6] Deininger MO, Moreira LFP, Dallan LAO, et al. Comparative analysis of the patency of the internal thoracic artery in the CABG of left anterior descending artery: 6-month postoperative coronary CT angiography evaluation. Revista Brasileira De Cirurgia Cardiovascular [online]. 2014;**29**: https://doi.org/10.5935/1678-9741.20140032

[7] Parsa CJ, Daneshmand MA, Gaca JG, et al. Arterial bypass grafting of the coronary circulation. HSR Proceedings in Intensive Care and Cardiovascular Anesthesia. 2011;**3**:227-234

[8] Brundage BH, Lipton MJ, Herfkens RJ, et al. Detection of patent artery bypass grafts by CT. Circulation. 1980;**61**:826-831 https://doi.org/10.1161/01.CIR.61.4.826

[9] Barbero U, Iannaccone M, d'Ascenzo F, et al. 64 slice-coronary computed tomography sensitivity and specificity in the evaluation of coronary artery bypass graft stenosis: A meta-analysis. International Journal of Cardiology. 2016;**216**:52 https://doi.org/10.1016/j.ijcard.2016.04.156

[10] Ropers D, Ulzheimer S, Orlov B, et al. Investigation of aortocoronary artery bypass grafts by multislice spiral CT with electrocardiographic—Gated image reconstruction. The American Journal of Cardiology. 2001;**88**:792-795 https://doi.org/10.1016/S0002-9149(01)01855-0

[11] Nieman K, Pattynama PM, Rensing BJ, et al. Evaluation of patients after coronary artery bypass surgery: CT angiographic assessment of grafts and coronary arteries. Radiology. 2003;**229**:749-756 https://doi.org/10.1148/radiol.2293020856

[12] Martuscelli E, Romagnoli A, D'Eliseo A, et al. Evaluation of venous and arterial conduit patency by 16-slice spiral CT. Circulation. 2004;**110**:3234-3238 https://doi.org/10.1161/01.CIR.0000147277.52036.07

[13] Schlosser T, Konorza T, Hunold P, et al. Noninvasive visualization of coronary artery bypass grafts using 16-detector row computed tomography. Journal of the American College of Cardiology. 2004;**44**:1224-1229 https://doi.org/10.1016/j.jacc.2003.09.075

[14] Hamon M, Lepage O, Malagutti P, et al. Diagnostic performance of 16 and 64 section spiral CT for coronary artery bypass grafts assessment. Radiology. 2008;**247**:679-686 https://doi.org/10.1148/radiol.2473071132

[15] Nazeri I, Shahabi P, Tehrai M, Sharif-Kashani B, Nazeri A. Assessment of patients after aortocoronary bypass grafting using 64-slice computed tomography. The American Journal of Cardiology. 2009;**103**:667-673 https://doi.org/10.1016/j.amjcard.2008.10.040

[16] Malagutti P, Nieman K, Meijboom WB, et al. Use of 64-slice CT in symptomatic patients after coronary bypass surgery: Evaluation of grafts and coronary arteries. European Heart Journal. 2007;**28**:1879-1885 https://doi.org/10.1093/eurheartj/ehl155

[17] Meyer TS, Martinoff S, Hadamitzky M, et al. Improved noninvasive assessment of coronary artery bypass grafts with 64-slice computed tomographic angiography in an unselected patient population. Journal of the American College of Cardiology. 2007;**49**:946-950 https://doi.org/10.1016/j.jacc.2006.10.066

[18] Locker C, Schaff HV, Dearani JA, Joyce LD, Park SJ, Burkhart HM, et al. Multiple arterial grafts improve late survival of patients undergoing coronary artery bypass graft surgery: Analysis of 8622 patients with multivessel disease. Circulation. 2012;**126**(9):1023-1030 https://doi.org/10.1161/CIRCULATIONAHA.111.084624

[19] Dewey M, Zimmermann E, Deissenrieder F, et al. Noninvasive coronary angiography by 320 row CT w th lower radiation exposure and maintained diagnostic accuracy. Circulation. 2009;**120**:867-875 https://doi.org/10.1161/CIRCULATIONAHA.109.859280

[20] Chao SP, Leu JG, Law WY, Kuo CJ, Shyu KG. Image quality of 256-slice computed tomography for coronary angiography. Acta Cardiologica Sinica. 2013;**29**:444-450. (print); ISSN 2375-7264 (online). http://www.jofamericanscience.org. 13. DOI: 10.7537/marsjas120816.13.

[21] Steigner M, Otero H, Mitsouras D, et al. Narrowing the phase window width in prospectively ECG gated single heart beat 320-detector row coronary CT angiography. The International Journal of Cardiovascular Imaging. 2009;**25**:85-89 https://doi.org/10.1007/s10554-008-9347-8

[22] Hendel RC, Patel MR, Kramer CM, et al. ACCF/ACR/SCCT/SCMR/ASNC/NASCI/SCAI/SIR 2006 appropriateness criteria for cardiac computed tomography and cardiac magnetic resonance imaging. Journal of the American College of Cardiology. 2006;**48**:1475-1497 https://doi.org/10.1016/j.jacc.2006.07.003

[23] Eisenberg C, Hulten E, Bittencourt MS, Blankstein R. Use of CT angiography among patients with prior coronary artery bypass grafting surgery. Cardiovascular Diagnosis and Therapy. 2017;**7**(1):102-105. DOI: 10.21037/cdt.2016.11.08

[24] Hermann F, Martinoff S, Meyer T, et al. Reduction of radiation estimates in cardiac 64-slice CT angiography in patients after coronary by artery bypass graft surgery. Investigative Radiology. 2008;**43**:253-260 https://doi.org/10.1097/RLI.0b013e318160b3a3

[25] Di Lazzaro D, Crusco F. CT angio for the evaluation of graft patency. Journal of Thoracic Disease. 2017;**9**(Suppl 4):S283-S288. DOI: 10.21037/jtd.2017.03.111

[26] Patra S, Jena M, Pande A, Ghosh D, Chakraborty RN. Assessment of coronary artery bypass grafts status in symptomatic patients: An observational study. The Journal of Cardiovascular Thoracic Surgery. 2017;**2**(1):4

[27] Hemat EM, Zidan EH, Ismail AA, Khalil WA. Multislice CT angiography assessment of coronary artery bypass graft (CABG) patients. Journal of American Science. 2016;**12**(8):92-98. ISSN 1545-1003 (print); ISSN 2375-7264 (online). http://www.jofamericanscience.org. 13. doi: 10.7537/marsjas120816.13

[28] Sundaram B, Quint LE, Patel HJ, Deeb GM. CT findings following thoracic aortic surgery. Radiographics. 2007;**27**:1583-1594 https://doi.org/10.1148/rg.276075004

[29] Onuma Y, Tanabe K, Chihara R, et al. Evaluation of coronary artery bypass grafts and native coronary arteries using 64-slice multidetector computed tomography. American Heart Journal. 2007;**154**:519-526 https://doi.org/10.1016/j.ahj.2007.04.054

[30] Cao C, Ang SC, Wolak K, Peeceeyen S, Bannon P, Yan TDA. Meta-analysis of randomized controlled trials on mid-term angiographic outcomes for radial artery versus saphenous vein in coronary artery bypass graft surgery. Annals of Cardiothoracic Surgery. 2013;**2**(4):401-407

[31] Bitkover CY, Cederlund K, Aberg B, Vaage J. Computed tomography of the sternum and mediastinum after median sternotomy. The Annals of Thoracic Surgery. 1999;**68**:858-863 https://doi.org/10.1016/S0003-4975(99)00549-4

[32] Pesenti-Rossi D, Baron N, Georges JL, et al. Assessment of coronary bypass graft patency by first-line multidetector computed tomography. Annales de Cardiologie et'd Angeiologie (Paris). 2014;**63**:284-292 https://doi.org/10.1016/j.ancard.2014.08.011

Chapter 2

The Choice of Graft Conduits in Coronary Artery Bypass Grafting

Takashi Murashita

Additional information is available at the end of the chapter

http://dx.doi.org/10.5772/intechopen.70398

Abstract

The use of the left internal mammary artery (IMA) has been shown to improve long-term survival and has been a gold standard in coronary artery bypass grafting (CABG). However, the choice of second or third graft conduit is still controversial. Multiple studies demonstrated the benefit of using multiple arterial grafts such as right IMA and radial artery in addition to left IMA in terms of long-term survival and graft patency. However, most of the centers still perform CABG with one IMA and vein grafts in a real world. The challenges for bilateral IMA utilization include longer operative time and concerns for higher rates of perioperative morbidity and mortality associated with increased sternal wound infection. Several studies reported that skeletonization technique can reduce the risk of sternal wound infection. Radial artery is another arterial conduit, which does not increase the risk of sternal wound infection and is easy to harvest. The superiority between radial artery and right IMA has been controversial. In the meantime, multiple trials have been made to improve the patency of vein grafts. The choice of graft conduits in CABG should be well considered preoperatively based on each patient's backgrounds.

Keywords: graft, conduit, coronary artery bypass grafting, internal mammary artery, greater saphenous vein, radial artery

1. Introduction

Coronary artery bypass grafting (CABG) is one of the most common operations performed in the United States [1], and it has been established as an effective treatment for severe coronary artery disease [2]. In fact, despite the increasing use of percutaneous coronary intervention (PCI) for coronary artery disease during the past decade [3], CABG remains the gold standard for multivessel coronary artery disease or left main disease [4, 5]. A number of major trials such as SYNTAX [6], ASCERT [7], and FREEDOM [8] reported superior long-term survival rates of CABG compared to PCI.

The main factor of the superiority of CABG over PCI is the use of internal mammary artery (IMA) to left anterior descending (LAD) artery [9, 10]. The excellent long-term patency of left IMA (LIMA) to LAD graft has been established [11–14] and the use of an IMA graft seems to improve long-term survival [15].

On the other hand, the long-term outcomes of other conduits such as saphenous vein graft, radial artery, and right gastroepiploic artery have been reported to be poorer than those of IMA. The patency rates of saphenous vein grafts were 71–87% at 1 year after surgery in previous studies [16–18] and up to 50% at 10 years [16–21].

Patients often require more than one bypass graft at the time of CABG. Unfortunately, there has been a lack of evidence for selecting bypass conduits beyond great confidence in the superiority of LIMA to LAD grafting. Therefore, the second best conduit for CABG is still unknown.

2. CABG with bilateral internal mammary arteries (BIMA)

2.1. Rationale for BIMA use

The advantages of arterial grafts over vein grafts include the inherent characteristics of the arterial endothelium of the left IMA graft [22–24]. The excellent long-term outcomes of single IMA graft have stimulated the use of a bilateral IMA approach [25]. A number of previous studies have reported the superiority of BIMA use over single IMA use (**Table 1**) [41–43].

Despite these evidences, BIMA use still appears to remain underutilized in the modern era. The challenges for BIMA utilization include longer operative time and concerns for higher rates of perioperative morbidity and mortality associated with increased sternal wound infection. LaPar and colleagues reviewed a total of 43,823 primary, isolated CABG patients in a Society of Thoracic Surgeons Database [44]. They found that the overall BIMA use was 3%, and even in low-risk patients, BIMA was used only in 6%. Importantly, BIMA use was not associated with increased postoperative mortality, morbidity, or hospital length of stay. However, hospital readmission rate was greater in BIMA patients compared with that in single IMA patients.

The configuration of BIMA grafts has also been controversial. Glineur et al. performed a prospective randomized trial that showed that the graft patency of BIMA grafts was similar between in-situ and Y-grafting configuration, whereas the use of BIMA in a Y-grafting configuration was associated in lower rates of major adverse cardiovascular and cerebrovascular events [45].

2.2. A randomized trial of BIMA use

A randomized trial of BIMA use for CABG, the arterial revascularization trial (ART) has been ongoing [46]. The patients were randomly scheduled for CABG to undergo single IMA or BIMA grafting in 28 cardiac surgical centers in 7 countries. A total of more than 3000 patients were enrolled in this study. Their results demonstrated no difference between single IMA use

Study	Year	Number of pts	Follow-up (years)	Key outcomes
Endo et al. [26]	2001	BIMA 443, SIMA 688	6.15	Graft patency was 97.3% in the BIMA group and 94.3% in the SIMA group ($p < 0.0001$).
Endo et al. [27]	2003	BIMA 190, SIMA 27	8.1	10-year survival rate was significantly better in BIMA group than in SIMA group (87.8 ± 3.5 vs 75.2 ± 3.4%, $p = 0.04$), and 10-year all death–free or repeat CABG or recurrent MI–free rate was significantly better in BIMA group than in SIMA group (86.6 ± 3.6 vs 69.0 ± 3.7%, $p = 0.0086$).
Lytle et al. [28]	2004	BIMA 2001, SIMA 8123	16.5	Survival of BIMA and SIMA groups at 7, 10, 15, and 20 years was 89 vs 87%, 81 vs 78%, 67 vs 58%, and 50 vs 37%, respectively ($p < 0.0001$).
Calafiore et al. [29]	2004	BIMA 1026, SIMA 576	7.3 ± 4.8	BIMA group had better freedom from cardiac death at 10 years (96.5 ± 0.8 vs 91.3 ± 1.4, $p = 0.0288$), late MI (98.0 ± 0.6 vs 94.3 ± 1.2, $p = 0.0180$), late MI in a grafted area (98.4 ± 0.6 vs 94.7 ± 1.1, $p = 0.0057$), and late cardiac events (93.9 ± 1.1 vs 86.3 ± 1.8, $p = 0.0388$).
Stevens et al. [30]	2005	BIMA 214, SIMA 419	11 ± 3	BIMA grafting decreased the risk of death (Hazard Ratio = 0.72 [0.57–0.91, 95% CI]) and coronary reoperation (HR = 0.38 [0.19–0.77]) in both diabetic and nondiabetic patients.
Di Mauro et al. [31]	2005	Matched; BIMA 476, SIMA 476	8.8 ± 4.0	BIMA group showed a better 10-year freedom from all-cause death (92.4 ± 2.1 vs 87.5 ± 3.5%, $p = 0.0216$), cardiac death (97.4 ± 0.9 vs 91.9 ± 1.4%, $p = 0.0042$), MI (98.7 ± 0.5 vs 94.2 ± 1.2%, $p = 0.0034$), MI in a grafted area (98.9 ± 0.5 vs 94.7 ± 1.3%, $p = 0.0017$), cardiac events (95.4 ± 1.2 vs 86.8 ± 1.8%, $p = 0.0026$), and any events (88.8 ± 2.2 vs 80.7 ± 2.1%, $p = 0.0124$).
Rankin et al. [32]	2007	BIMA 377, SIMA 490	up to 20 years	The composite of mortality, MI, PCI, and redo CABG was lower in BIMA group than in SIMA group ($p = 0.013$).
Mohammadi et al. [33]	2008	BIMA 1338, SIMA 9566	5.7 ± 3.7	Survival rates at 5, 7, and 10 years were 98.4, 97.8, and 96.5%, respectively, for patients with BIMA use, which were significantly higher ($p < 0.0001$) compared to the patients with SIMA use (96.6, 94.3, and 88.9%, respectively).
Kurlansky et al. [34]	2010	BIMA 2215, SIMA 2369	11.1–12.7	At 15 years, survival for SIMA and BIMA patients was 37.5 ± 1.1% and 53.5 ± 1.2%, respectively; at 25 years, it was 15.7 ± 2.0% for SIMA patients and 28.6 ± 2.2% for BIMA patients ($p < 0.001$).
Kieser et al. [35]	2011	BIMA 1038, SIMA 4029	7.1	Patients undergoing BIMA grafting had the lowest 1-year mortality (2.4 vs 4.3% SIMA grafting and 8.2% vein-only grafting; $p < 0.0001$).
Grau et al. [36]	2012	Matched; BIMA 928 and SIMA 928	9.0 ± 5	10-year survival for BIMA was 89% and for LIMA was 79% ($p < 0.001$).

Study	Year	Number of pts	Follow-up (years)	Key outcomes
Galbut et al. [37]	2012	Matched; BIMA 87 and SIMA 87 in EF < 30% group, BIMA 448 and SIMA 448 in EF 30–50% group, BIMA 1137 and SIMA 1137 in EF > 50% group	7.0–13	10- and 20-year survival, SIMA vs BIMA, in EF 30–50% group was 57.7 ± 0.3 and 19 ± 2.5 vs 62.0 ± 2.3 and 33.1 ± 3.4%, respectively, $p = 0.016$; and in EF > 50% group, it was 67.1 ± 1.4 and 35.8 ± 1.7 vs 74.6 ± 1.3 and 38.1 ± 2.1%, respectively, $p = 0.012$.
Locker et al. [38]	2012	BIMA/SVG 589, BIMA only 271, BIMA-RA 147, LIMA/SVG 7435	7.6 ± 4.6	BIMA/SVG and BIMA only had improved survival (86 and 76%; 82 and 75% at 10 and 15 years [$p < 0.001$]), and patients with BIMA/RA and LIMA/RA had greater 10-year survival (84 and 78%; $p < 0.001$) vs LIMA/SVG.
Kinoshita et al. [39]	2012	BIMA 244, SIMA 247	4.3 ± 1.6	The 5-year estimated freedom rate from overall death and cardiac event was higher in the BIMA group than in the SIMA group: 86.4 ± 3.2 vs 73.5 ± 3.9% ($p = 0.01$) and 93.2 ± 2.7 vs 87.5 ± 3.0% ($p = 0.01$), respectively.
Puskas et al. [40]	2012	BIMA 812, SIMA 2715	n.a.	BIMA was associated with a significant overall survival advantage at 8 years of follow-up of 89.3% compared with 68.3% with use of SIMA ($p < 0.001$).

MI, myocardial infarction; PCI, percutaneous coronary intervention; CABG, coronary artery bypass grafting; EF, ejection fraction; SVG, saphenous vein graft; RA, radial artery.

Table 1. Previous studies that reported the superiority of bilateral internal mammary artery (BIMA) use over single internal mammary artery (SIMA) use.

and BIMA use in terms of mortality or the rates of cardiovascular events at 5 years of follow-up [47]. Rates of major bleeding events and the need for repeat revascularization, angina status, and quality-of-life measures did not differ between the two groups, either. On the other hand, there were more sternal wound complications with BIMA use than with single IMA use. The ten-year outcomes are pending.

2.3. Sternal wound infection

One of the reasons of reluctant use of BIMA is a concern for potential sternal wound infection. There are basically two techniques for harvesting IMA: pedicled and skeletonized. Harvesting an ITA with a pedicled fashion can potentially lead to sternal devascularisation; however, Kamiya et al. reported that the damage can be minimized with skeletonization by preserving sternal and intercostal branches of IMA [48]. Boodhwani et al. reported that skeletonization resulted in reduced postoperative pain and increased sternal perfusion [49]. However, skeletonization is more technically demanding and time-consuming, and there is a concern of increased risk of injury of IMA during harvesting. Therefore, there is still a controversy regarding superiority between the two techniques.

Several previous studies reported that the skeletonization technique has a benefit over pedicled technique in terms of the incidence of sternal wound complication. Benedetto et al. reported that the risk of sternal wound infection was similar between skeletonized BIMA and pedicled single IMA [50]. Kai et al. reported that off-pump CABG with skeletonized BMA use resulted in a low incidence of sternal wound infection (0.6%) even in insulin-dependent diabetes patients [51].

3. CABG using radial artery graft

Due to the complexity of BIMA use, radial artery (RA) has been a preferred arterial graft over right IMA. RA is easier to harvest than IMA and not associated with sternal wound infection. Multiple previous studies reported improved long-term survival and patency rates for patients receiving RA as a second arterial graft compared with patients receiving vein grafts only [52–55].

However, RA is muscular and vulnerable to spasm and competitive flow. A previous study reported that the lower capacity of nitric oxide release may contribute to the susceptibility of RA to the vasospasm and may have an impact on the long-term patency [56].

There is a big controversy about which is the second best arterial graft between RA and right IMA [57] (**Table 2**). Tranbaugh et al. conducted a propensity matched study comparing RA and right IMA grafts to bypass the left circumflex coronary artery [58]. They concluded RA had fewer major adverse events, a similar patency to right IMA, and improved survival in older and chronic obstructive pulmonary disease patients. Caputo et al. reported that RA provided better early and mid-term outcomes compared to right IMA [59].

Study	Year	Number of pts	Survival	Graft patency	Conclusions
Tranbaugh et al. [58]	2014	Matched 528	10 year: 85% for RA and 80% for RIMA ($p = 0.060$)	83.9% for RA and 87.4% for RIMA at 5.1 ± 3.8 years ($p = 0.155$)	RA > RIMA
Caputo et al. [59]	2003	325 for RA, 336 for RIMA	18 months: 99.7% for RA and 98.4% for RIMA ($p = 0.07$)	n.a.	RA > RIMA
Hayward et al. [60]	2007	198 for RA, 196 for RIMA	Mean of 6.0 years follow-up: 13 deaths in RA and 18 deaths in RIMA ($p = 0.36$)	n.a.	RA = RIMA
Hayward et al. [61]	2010	198 for RA, 196 for RIMA	n.a.	5-years; 89.8% for RA, 83.2% for RIMA ($p = 0.06$)	RA = RIMA
Ruttman et al. [62]	2011	724 for RA, 277 for RIMA	5 years: 93.0% for RA and 98.9% for RIMA ($p = 0.022$)	RA occlusion was found in 37.9%; IMA occlusion was found in 10.2% ($p < 0.001$)	RA < RIMA
Raja et al. [63]	2015	Matched; 779 for RA and 747 for RIMA	10 years: 87.8% for RA and 93.4% for RIMA ($p = -0.008$)	n.a.	RA < RIMA

Table 2. Previous studies that compared right internal mammary artery (RIMA) and radial artery (RA).

Hayward et al. conducted a randomized study and concluded that, when patients receive a left IMA graft to the LAD, the next target may be grafted with a RA or a free right IMA to achieve similar clinical outcomes based on a mean of 6-year follow-up [60]. To the contrary, Ruttman et al. reported a superiority of right IMA graft compared to RA in terms of both survival and cardiac-related morbidity [62]. Raja et al. also reported the superiority of RIMA over RA [63].

4. CABG using saphenous vein grafts

Despite the potential benefits of multiple arterial grafts [41], saphenous vein graft (SVG) is still the most frequently used conduit in CABG. However, the long-term patency of SVG is reported to be poor [16–21]. The late-term SVG failure is mainly due to atherosclerotic obstruction occurring on a foundation of neointimal hyperplasia [64]. Attempts to mitigate intimal hyperplasia and SVG failure have been made; however, only persistent use of statin therapy and beta-blockers have been shown to reduce intimal hyperplasia in vein grafts [65]. Edifoligide [16] and aspirin plus clopidogrel have failed to reduce the process of SVG intimal hyperplasia [66].

Mechanical external stenting with polyester has shown potential benefits in preclinical testing with reduction of both neointima formation and early atherosclerosis, both of which are key aspects of SVG disease [67, 68]. The outcomes of initial trials of external stents for SVG were poor. Murphy et al. reported 100% occlusion of external stented SVG at 6 months [69]. Schoettler et al. reported that the patency rate of mesh-supported SVG was 27.8% at 9 months, whereas conventional SVG showed 85.7% patency [70]. Rescigno et al. reported 66.9% occlusion at 12 months of SVG supported with nitinol mesh [71]. Taggart et al. performed a randomized study comparing the one-year patency rate of stented SVG vs nonstented SVG [72]. They reported that the overall SVG failure rates did not differ between the stented SVG and nonstented SVG (30 vs 28.2%); however, stented SVG had less intimal hyperplasia and better lumen uniformity.

On the other hand, a previous study showed that the "nontouch technique," in which SVG is harvested with a pedicle of surrounding tissue, was associated with a decreased vascular smooth muscle cell activation, which affects long-term patency of SVG [73]. Souza et al. conducted a randomized study comparing graft patency of SVGs using nontouch technique and those using conventional technique [74]. They concluded that harvesting SVG with surrounding tissue provided excellent short- and long-term patency, which was comparable to the IMA [75].

5. CABG using right gastroepiploic artery

The successful use of right gastroepiploic artery (GEA) in CABG was reported in 1980s [76–78]. Histologically, GEA contains many smooth muscle cells in the media, whereas IMA has rich elastic fibers in the media [79]. Therefore, GEA is considered as a muscular artery, whereas IMA is an elastic artery. This difference becomes important when harvesting a graft, because GEA is more vulnerable to spasm than IMA.

GEA is most suitable for grafting to the distal right coronary artery and the posterior descending artery because this site is the nearest for the in-situ GEA graft and the most distant from the in-situ right IMA graft. In addition, in-situ GEA grafting can avoid manipulation of the aorta and can result in less neurological complications [80, 81].

Suma et al. reported that the cumulative patency rate of GEA graft was 92.3% at 1 year, 85.5% at 5 years, and 66.5% at 10 years after surgery, and skeletonization technique can improve the graft patency [82]. Suzuki et al. reported that skeletonized GEA grafting to the right coronary artery provided better survival and lower adverse cardiac events than SVG grafting [83].

In a real world, although multiple studies also demonstrated excellent surgical outcomes of CABG using GEA graft [84–87], GEA is rarely used in the United States mainly due to technical complexity.

6. Conclusions

CABG has been a gold standard for severe multivessel coronary artery disease. There is a conclusive evidence of a benefit of using IMA in CABG surgery. Therefore, arterial grafts are thought to provide better outcomes than vein grafts. In a real world, however, multiple arterial revascularization is still underutilized. There are multiple studies that showed a survival benefit of using right IMA or radial artery as a second arterial graft compared to using vein grafts. The superiority of right IMA vs radial artery is still controversial. Some studies suggested skeletonization technique can minimize the risk of sternal wound infection, which is the main concern for using bilateral IMAs. In the meantime, multiple trials or techniques have been tried to improve the long-term patency of vein grafts.

Author details

Takashi Murashita

Address all correspondence to: tmurashita@gmail.com

Heart and Vascular Institute, West Virginia University, Morgantown, WV, USA

References

[1] ElBardissi A, Aranki S, Sheng S, O'Brien S, Greenberg C, Gammie J. Trends in isolated coronary artery bypass grafting: An analysis of the Society of Thoracic Surgeons adult

cardiac surgery database. Journal of Thoracic and Cardiovascular Surgery 2012;**143**:273-281. DOI: 10.1016/j.jtcvs.2011.10.029

[2] Yusuf S, Zucker D, Peduzzi P, Fisher L, Takaro T, Kennedy J, Davis K, Killip T, Passamani E, Norris R. Effect of coronary artery bypass graft surgery on survival: Overview of 10-year results from randomised trials by the Coronary Artery Bypass Graft Surgery Trialists Collaboration. Lancet 1994;**344**:563-570.

[3] Epstein AJ, Polsky D, Yang F, Yang L, Groeneveld PW. Coronary revascularization trends in the United States, 2001-2008. Journal of the American Medical Association 2011;**305**:1769-1776. DOI: 10.1001/jama.2011.551

[4] Serruys PW, Morice MC, Kappetein AP, Colombo A, Holmes DR, Mack MJ, Ståhle E, Feldman TE, van den Brand M, Bass EJ, Van Dyck N, Leadley K, Dawkins KD, Mohr FW, SYNTAX Investigators. Percutaneous coronary intervention versus coronary-artery bypass grafting for severe coronary artery disease. New England Journal of Medicine 2009;**360**:961-972. DOI: 10.1056/NEJMoa0804626

[5] Benedetto U, Gaudino M, Ng C, Biondi-Zoccai G, D'Ascenzo F, Frati G, Girardi L, Angelini G, Taggart D. Coronary surgery is superior to drug eluting stents in multivessel disease. Systematic review and meta-analysis of contemporary randomized controlled trials. International Journal of Cardiology. 2016;**210**:19-24. DOI: 10.1016/j.ijcard.2016.02.090

[6] Mohr FW, Morice MC, Kappetein AP, Feldman TE, Ståhle E, Colombo A, Mack MJ, Holmes DR, Jr., Morel MA, Van Dyck N, Houle VM, Dawkins KD, Serruys PW. Coronary artery bypass graft surgery versus percutaneous coronary intervention in patients with three-vessel disease and left main coronary disease: 5-year follow-up of the randomised, clinical SYNTAX trial. Lancet 2013;**381**:629-638. DOI: 10.1016/S0140-6736(13)60141-5

[7] Weintraub WS, Grau-Sepulveda MV, Weiss JM, O'Brien SM, Peterson ED, Kolm P, Zhang Z, Klein LW, Shaw RE, McKay C, Ritzenthaler LL, Popma JJ, Messenger JC, Shahian DM, Grover FL, Mayer JE, Shewan CM, Garratt KN, Moussa ID, Dangas GD, Edwards FH. Comparative effectiveness of revascularization strategies. New England Journal of Medicine. 2012;**366**:1467-1476. DOI: 10.1056/NEJMoa1110717

[8] Farkouh ME, Domanski M, Sleeper LA, Siami FS, Dangas G, Mack M, Yang M, Cohen DJ, Rosenberg Y, Solomon SD, Desai AS, Gersh BJ, Magnuson EA, Lansky A, Boineau R, Weinberger J, Ramanathan K, Sousa JE, Rankin J, Bhargava B, Buse J, Hueb W, Smith CR, Muratov V, Bansilal S, King S, 3rd., Bertrand M, Fuster V, FREEDOM Trial Investigators. Strategies for multivessel revascularization in patients with diabetes. New England Journal of Medicine 2012;**367**:2375-2384. DOI: 10.1056/NEJMoa1211585

[9] Wrigley BJ, Dubey G, Spyt T, Gershlick AH. Hybrid revascularisation in multivessel coronary artery disease: Could a combination of CABG and PCI be the best option in selected patients? EuroIntervention 2013;**8**:1335-1341. DOI:10.4244/EIJV8I11A202

[10] Harskamp RE, Zheng Z, Alexander JH, Williams JB, Xian Y, Halkos ME, Brennan JM, de Winter RJ, Smith PK, Lopes RD. Status quo of hybrid coronary revascularization for multi-vessel coronary artery disease. Annals of Thoracic Surgery 2013;**96**:2268-2277.

[11] Shah PJ, Durairaj M, Gordon I, Fuller J, Rosalion A, Seevanayagam S, Tatoulis J, Buxton BF. Factors affecting patency of internal thoracic artery graft: Clinical and angiographic study in 1434 symptomatic patients operated between 1982 and 2002. European Journal of Cardio-Thoracic Surgery 2004;**26**:118-124. DOI: 10.1016/j.ejcts.2004.02.037

[12] Cameron A, Davis KB, Green G, Schaff HV. Coronary bypass surgery with internal-thoracic-artery grafts--effects on survival over a 15-year period. New England Journal of Medicine. 1996;**334**:216-219. DOI: 10.1056/NEJM199601253340402

[13] Loop FD, Lytle BW, Cosgrove DM, Stewart RW, Goormastic M, Williams GW, Golding LA, Gill CC, Taylor PC, Sheldon WC. Influence of the internal-mammary-artery graft on 10-year survival and other cardiac events. New England Journal of Medicine. 1986;**314**:1-6. DOI: 10.1056/NEJM198601023140101

[14] Cameron A, Green G, Brogno D, Thornton J. Internal thoracic artery grafts: 20-year clinical follow-up. Journal of the American College of Cardiology. 1995;**25**:188-192

[15] Hlatky M, Shilane D, Boothroyd D, Boersma E, Brooks M, Carrié D, Clayton T, Danchin N, Flather M, Hamm C, Hueb W, Kahler J, Lopes N, Pocock S, Rodriguez A, Serruys P, Sigwart U, Stables R. The effect of internal thoracic artery grafts on long-term clinical outcomes after coronary bypass surgery. Journal of Thoracic and Cardiovascular Surgery. 2011;**142**:829-835. DOI: 10.1016/j.jtcvs.2010.09.063

[16] Alexander JH, Hafley G, Harrington RA, Peterson ED, Ferguson TB, Jr., Lorenz TJ, Goyal A, Gibson M, Mack MJ, Gennevois D, Califf RM, Kouchoukos NT, PREVENT IV Investigators. Efficacy and safety of edifoligide, an E2F transcription factor decoy, for prevention of vein graft failure following coronary artery bypass graft surgery: PREVENT IV: A randomized controlled trial. Journal of the American Medical Association. 2005;**294**:2446-2454. DOI: 10.1001/jama.294.19.2446

[17] Harskamp RE, Lopes RD, Baisden CE, de Winter RJ, Alexander JH. Saphenous vein graft failure after coronary artery bypass surgery: Pathophysiology, management, and future directions. Annals of Surgery 2013;**257**:824-833. DOI: 10.1097/SLA.0b013e318288c38d

[18] Puskas JD, Williams WH, Mahoney EM, Huber PR, Block PC, Duke PG, Staples JR, Glas KE, Marshall JJ, Leimbach ME, McCall SA, Petersen RJ, Bailey DE, Weintraub WS, Guyton RA. Off-pump vs conventional coronary artery bypass grafting: Early and 1-year graft patency, cost, and quality-of-life outcomes: A randomized trial. Journal of the American Medical Association 2004;**291**:1841-1849. DOI: 10.1001/jama.291.15.1841

[19] Tatoulis J, Buxton BF, Fuller JA. Patencies of 2127 arterial to coronary conduits over 15 years. Annals of Thoracic Surgery. 2004;**77**:93-101

[20] Goldman S, Zadina K, Moritz T, Ovitt T, Sethi G, Copeland JG, Thottapurathu L, Krasnicka B, Ellis N, Anderson RJ, Henderson W, VA Cooperative Study Group. Long-term patency of saphenous vein and left internal mammary artery grafts after coronary artery bypass surgery: Results from a Department of Veterans Affairs Cooperative Study. Journal of the American College of Cardiology 2004;**44**:2149-2156. DOI: 10.1016/j.jacc.2004.08.064

[21] Fitzgibbon G, Kafka H, Leach A, Keon W, Hooper G, Burton J. Coronary bypass graft fate and patient outcome: Angiographic follow-up of 5065 grafts related to survival and reoperation in 1388 patients during 25 years. Journal of the American College of Cardiology 1996;**28**:616-626.

[22] Glineur D, Poncelet A, El Khoury G, D'hoore W, Astarci P, Zech F, Noirhomme P, Hanet C. Fractional flow reserve of pedicled internal thoracic artery and saphenous vein grafts 6 months after bypass surgery. European Journal of Cardio-Thoracic Surgery. 2007;**31**:376-381. DOI: 10.1016/j.ejcts.2006.11.023

[23] Gurné O, Chenu P, Buche M, Louagie Y, Eucher P, Marchandise B, Rombaut E, Blommaert D, Schroeder E. Adaptive mechanisms of arterial and venous coronary bypass grafts to an increase in flow demand. Heart. 1999;**82**:336-342

[24] Walpoth B, Schmid M, Schwab A, Bosshard A, Eckstein F, Carrel T, Hess O. Vascular adaptation of the internal thoracic artery graft early and late after bypass surgery. Journal of Thoracic and Cardiovascular Surgery. 2008;**136**:876-883. DOI: 10.1016/j.jtcvs.2008.05.029

[25] Glineur D, Papadatos S, Grau J, Shaw R, Kuschner C, Aphram G, Mairy Y, Vanbelighen C, Etienne P. Complete myocardial revascularization using only bilateral internal thoracic arteries provides a low-risk and durable 10-year clinical outcome. European Journal of Cardio-Thoracic Surgery. 2016;**50**:735-741. DOI: 10.1016/j.ejcts.2004.01.001

[26] Endo M, Nishida H, Tomizawa Y, Kasanuki H. Benefit of bilateral over single internal mammary artery grafts for multiple coronary artery bypass grafting. Circulation. 2001;**104**:2164-2170

[27] Endo M, Tomizawa Y, Nishida H. Bilateral versus unilateral internal mammary revascularization in patients with diabetes. Circulation. 2003;**108**:1343-1349. DOI: 10.1161/01.CIR.0000085995.87982.6E

[28] Lytle B, Blackstone E, Sabik J, Houghtaling P, Loop F, Cosgrove D. The effect of bilateral internal thoracic artery grafting on survival during 20 postoperative years. Annals of Thoracic Surgery. 2004;**78**:2005-2012. DOI: 10.1016/j.athoracsur.2004.05.070

[29] Calafiore A, Di Giammarco G, Teodori G, Di Mauro M, Iacò A, Bivona A, Contini M, Vitolla G. Late results of first myocardial revascularization in multiple vessel disease: Single versus bilateral internal mammary artery with or without saphenous vein grafts. European Journal of Cardio-Thoracic Surgery 2004;**26**:542-548. DOI: 10.1016/j.ejcts.2004.05.028

[30] Stevens L, Carrier M, Perrault L, Hébert Y, Cartier R, Bouchard D, Fortier A, Pellerin M. Influence of diabetes and bilateral internal thoracic artery grafts on long-term outcome for multivessel coronary artery bypass grafting. European Journal of Cardio-Thoracic Surgery. 2005;**27**:281-288. DOI: 10.1016/j.ejcts.2004.10.048

[31] Di Mauro M, Iacò A, Contini M, Vitolla G, Weltert L, Di Giammarco G, Calafiore A. First time myocardial revascularization in patients younger than 70 years. Single versus double internal mammary artery. Italian Heart Journal. 2005;**6**:390-395

[32] Rankin J, Tuttle R, Wechsler A, Teichmann T, Glower D, Califf R. Techniques and benefits of multiple internal mammary artery bypass at 20 years of follow-up. Annals of Thoracic Surgery. 2007;**83**:1008-1014. DOI: 10.1016/j.athoracsur.2006.10.032

[33] Mohammadi S, Dagenais F, Doyle D, Mathieu P, Baillot R, Charbonneau E, Perron J, Voisine P. Age cut-off for the loss of benefit from bilateral internal thoracic artery grafting. European Journal of Cardio-Thoracic Surgery. 2008;**33**:977-982. DOI: 10.1016/j.ejcts.2008.03.026

[34] Kurlansky P, Traad E, Dorman M, Galbut D, Zucker M, Ebra G. Thirty-year follow-up defines survival benefit for second internal mammary artery in propensity-matched groups. Annals of Thoracic Surgery. 2010;**90**:101-108. DOI: 10.1016/j.athoracsur.2010.04.006

[35] Kieser T, Lewin A, Graham M, Martin B, Galbraith P, Rabi D, Norris C, Faris P, Knudtson M, Ghali W, APPROACH Investigators. Outcomes associated with bilateral internal thoracic artery grafting: The importance of age. Annals of Thoracic Surgery. 2011;**92**:1269-1275. DOI: 10.1016/j.athoracsur.2011.05.083

[36] Grau J, Ferrari G, Mak A, Shaw R, Brizzio M, Mindich B, Strobeck J, Zapolanski A. Propensity matched analysis of bilateral internal mammary artery versus single left internal mammary artery grafting at 17-year follow-up: Validation of a contemporary surgical experience. European Journal of Cardio-Thoracic Surgery 2012;**41**:770-775. DOI: 10.1093/ejcts/ezr213

[37] Galbut D, Kurlansky P, Traad E, Dorman M, Zucker M, Ebra G. Bilateral internal thoracic artery grafting improves long-term survival in patients with reduced ejection fraction: A propensity-matched study with 30-year follow-up. Journal of Thoracic and Cardiovascular Surgery. 2012;**143**:844-853. DOI: 10.1016/j.jtcvs.2011.12.026

[38] Locker C, Schaff H, Dearani J, Joyce L, Park S, Burkhart H, Suri R, Greason K, Stulak J, Li Z, Daly R. Multiple arterial grafts improve late survival of patients undergoing coronary artery bypass graft surgery: Analysis of 8622 patients with multivessel disease. Circulation 2012;**126**:1023-1030. DOI: 10.1161/CIRCULATIONAHA.111.084624

[39] Kinoshita T, Asai T, Suzuki T, Kuroyanagi S, Hosoba S, Takashima N. Off-pump bilateral skeletonized internal thoracic artery grafting in elderly patients. Annals of Thoracic Surgery. 2012;**93**:531-536. DOI: 10.1016/j.athoracsur.2011.09.077

[40] Puskas J, Sadiq A, Vassiliades T, Kilgo P, Lattouf O. Bilateral internal thoracic artery grafting is associated with significantly improved long-term survival, even among diabetic patients. Annals of Thoracic Surgery. 2012;**94**:710-715. DOI: 10.1016/j.athoracsur.2012.03.082

[41] Taggart D, D'Amico R, Altman D. Effect of arterial revascularisation on survival: A systematic review of studies comparing bilateral and single internal mammary arteries. Lancet 2001;**358**:870-875. DOI: 10.1016/S0140-6736(01)06069-X

[42] Yi G, Shine B, Rehman S, Altman D, Taggart D. Effect of bilateral internal mammary artery grafts on long-term survival: A meta-analysis approach. Circulation 2014;**130**:539-545. DOI: 10.1161/CIRCULATIONAHA.113.004255

[43] Smith T, Kloppenburg G, Morshuis W. Does the use of bilateral mammary artery grafts compared with the use of a single mammary artery graft offer a long-term survival benefit in patients undergoing coronary artery bypass surgery? Interactive Cardiovascular and Thoracic Surgery. 2014;**18**:96-101. DOI: 10.1093/icvts/ivt423

[44] LaPar D, Crosby I, Rich J, Quader M, Speir A, Kern J, Tribble C, Kron I, Ailawadi G, Investigators for the Virginia Cardiac Surgery Quality Initiative. Bilateral internal mammary artery use for coronary artery bypass grafting remains underutilized: A propensity-matched multi-institution analysis. Annals of Thoracic Surgery 2015;**100**:8-14. DOI: 10.1016/j.athoracsur.2015.02.088

[45] Glineur D, Boodhwani M, Hanet C, de Kerchove L, Navarra E, Astarci P, Noirhomme P, El Khoury G. Bilateral internal thoracic artery configuration for coronary artery bypass surgery: A prospective randomized trial. Circulation Cardiovascular Interventions. 2016;**9**:7. DOI: 10.1161/CIRCINTERVENTIONS.115.003518

[46] Taggart D, Altman D, Gray A, Lees B, Nugara F, Yu L, Campbell H, Flather M, ART Investigators. Randomized trial to compare bilateral vs. single internal mammary coronary artery bypass grafting: 1-year results of the Arterial Revascularisation Trial (ART). European Heart Journal. 2013;**31**:2470-2481. DOI: 10.1093/eurheartj/ehq318

[47] Taggart D, Altman D, Gray A, Lees B, Gerry S, Benedetto U, Flather M, ART Investigators. Randomized trial of bilateral versus single internal-thoracic-artery grafts. New England Journal of Medicine 2016;**375**:2540-2549. DOI: 10.1056/NEJMoa1610021

[48] Kamiya H, Akhyari P, Martens A, Karck M, Haverich A, Lichtenberg A. Sternal microcirculation after skeletonized versus pedicled harvesting of the internal thoracic artery: A randomized study. Journal of Thoracic and Cardiovascular Surgery 2008;**135**:32-37. DOI: 10.1016/j.jtcvs.2007.09.004

[49] Boodhwani M, Lam B, Nathan H, Mesana T, Ruel M, Zeng W, Sellke F, Rubens F. Skeletonized internal thoracic artery harvest reduces pain and dysesthesia and improves sternal perfusion after coronary artery bypass surgery: A randomized, double-blind, within-patient comparison. Circulation 2006;**114**:766-773. DOI:10.1161/CIRCULATIONAHA.106.615427

[50] Benedetto U, Altman D, Gerry S, Gray A, Lees B, Pawlaczyk R, Flather M, Taggart D, Arterial Revascularization Trial Investigators. Pedicled and skeletonized single and bilateral internal thoracic artery grafts and the incidence of sternal wound complications: Insights from the Arterial Revascularization Trial. Journal of Thoracic and Cardiovascular Surgery. 2016;**152**:270-276. DOI: 10.1016/j.jtcvs.2016.03.056

[51] Kai M, Hanyu M, Soga Y, Nomoto T, Nakano J, Matsuo T, Umehara E, Kawato M, Okabayashi H. Off-pump coronary artery bypass grafting with skeletonized bilateral internal thoracic arteries in insulin-dependent diabetics. Annals of Thoracic Surgery. 2007;**84**:32-36. DOI: 10.1016/j.athoracsur.2007.02.095

[52] Zacharias A, Habib R, Schwann T, Riordan C, Durham S, Shah A. Improved survival with radial artery versus vein conduits in coronary bypass surgery with left internal thoracic

artery to left anterior descending artery grafting. Circulation. 2004;**109**:1489-1496. DOI: 10.1161/01.CIR.0000121743.10146.78

[53] Collins P, Webb C, Chong C, Moat N, Radial Artery Versus Saphenous Vein Patency (RSVP) Trial Investigators. Radial artery versus saphenous vein patency randomized trial: Five-year angiographic follow-up. Circulation 2008;**117**:2859-2864. DOI: 10.1161/CIRCULATIONAHA.107.736215

[54] Tranbaugh R, Dimitrova K, Friedmann P, Geller C, Harris L, Stelzer P, Cohen B, Hoffman D. Radial artery conduits improve long-term survival after coronary artery bypass grafting. Annals of Thoracic Surgery. 2010;**90**:1165-1172. DOI: 10.1016/j.athoracsur.2010.05.038

[55] Schwann T, Tranbaugh R, Dimitrova K, Engoren M, Kabour A, Hoffman D, Geller C, Ko W, Habib R. Time-varying survival benefit of radial artery versus vein grafting: A multiinstitutional analysis. Annals of Thoracic Surgery 2014;**97**:1328-1334. DOI: 10.1016/j.athoracsur.2014.09.078

[56] He G, Liu Z. Comparison of nitric oxide release and endothelium-derived hyperpolarizing factor-mediated hyperpolarization between human radial and internal mammary arteries. Circulation. 2001;**104**:1344-1349

[57] Tatoulis J. Total arterial coronary revascularization-patient selection, stenoses, conduits, targets. Annals of Cardiothoracic Surgery. 2013;**2**:499-506. DOI: 10.3978/j.issn.2225-319X.2013.07.02

[58] Tranbaugh R, Dimitrova K, Lucido D, Hoffman D, Dincheva G, Geller C, Balaram S, Ko W, Swistel D. The second best arterial graft: A propensity analysis of the radial artery versus the free right internal thoracic artery to bypass the circumflex coronary artery. Journal of Thoracic and Cardiovascular Surgery 2014;**147**:133-140. DOI: 10.1016/j.jtcvs.2013.08.040

[59] Caputo M, Reeves B, Marchetto G, Mahesh B, Lim K, Angelini G. Radial versus right internal thoracic artery as a second arterial conduit for coronary surgery: Early and midterm outcomes. Journal of Thoracic and Cardiovascular Surgery 2003;**126**:39-47

[60] Hayward P, Hare D, Gordon I, Matalanis G, Buxton B. Which arterial conduit? Radial artery versus free right internal thoracic artery: Six-year clinical results of a randomized controlled trial. Annals of Thoracic Surgery 2007;**84**:493-497. DOI: 10.1016/j.athoracsur.2007.03.053

[61] Hayward P, Gordon I, Hare D, Matalanis G, Horrigan M, Rosalion A, Buxton B. Comparable patencies of the radial artery and right internal thoracic artery or saphenous vein beyond 5 years: Results from the Radial Artery Patency and Clinical Outcomes trial. Journal of Thoracic and Cardiovascular Surgery. 2010;**139**:60-65. DOI: 10.1016/j.jtcvs.2009.09.043

[62] Ruttmann E, Fischler N, Sakic A, Chevtchik O, Alber H, Schistek R, Ulmer H, Grimm M. Second internal thoracic artery versus radial artery in coronary artery bypass grafting: A long-term, propensity score-matched follow-up study. Circulation 2011;**124**:1321-1329. DOI: 10.1161/CIRCULATIONAHA.111.030536

[63] Raja S, Benedetto U, Jothidasan A, Jujjavarapu R, Ukwu U, De Robertis F, Bahrami T, Gaer J, Amrani M, Harefield Cardiac Outcomes Research Group. Right internal mammary artery versus radial artery as second arterial conduit in coronary artery bypass grafting: A case-control study of 1526 patients. International Journal of Surgery. 2015;**16**:183-189. DOI: 10.1016/j.ijsu.2014.08.342

[64] Motwani J, Topol E. Aortocoronary saphenous vein graft disease: Pathogenesis, predisposition, and prevention. Circulation 1998;**97**:916-931

[65] Une D, Kulik A, Voisine P, Le May M, Ruel M. Correlates of saphenous vein graft hyperplasia and occlusion 1 year after coronary artery bypass grafting: Analysis from the CASCADE randomized trial. Circulation 2013;**128**:S213-S218 DOI: 10.1161/CIRCULATIONAHA.112.000328

[66] Kulik A, Le May M, Voisine P, Tardif J, Delarochelliere R, Naidoo S, Wells G, Mesana T, Ruel M. Aspirin plus clopidogrel versus aspirin alone after coronary artery bypass grafting: The clopidogrel after surgery for coronary artery disease (CASCADE) Trial. Circulation. 2010;**122**:2680-2687. DOI: 10.1161/CIRCULATIONAHA.110.978007

[67] Angelini G, Lloyd C, Bush R, Johnson J, Newby A. An external, oversized, porous polyester stent reduces vein graft neointima formation, cholesterol concentration, and vascular cell adhesion molecule 1 expression in cholesterol-fed pigs. Journal of Thoracic and Cardiovascular Surgery. 2002;**124**:950-956

[68] Ben-Gal Y, Taggart D, Williams M, Orion E, Uretzky G, Shofti R, Banai S, Yosef L, Bolotin G. Expandable external support device to improve Saphenous Vein Graft Patency after CABG. Journal of Cardiothoracic Surgery 2013;**8**:122. DOI: 10.1186/1749-8090-8-122

[69] Murphy G, Newby A, Jeremy J, Baumbach A, Angelini G. A randomized trial of an external Dacron sheath for the prevention of vein graft disease: The Extent study. Journal of Thoracic and Cardiovascular Surgery 2007;**134**:504-505. DOI: 10.1016/j.jtcvs.2007.01.092

[70] Schoettler J, Jussli-Melchers J, Grothusen C, Stracke L, Schoeneich F, Stohn S, Hoffmann G, Cremer J. Highly flexible nitinol mesh to encase aortocoronary saphenous vein grafts: First clinical experiences and angiographic results nine months postoperatively. Interactive Cardiovascular and Thoracic Surgery 2011;**13**:396-400. DOI: 10.1510/icvts.2010.265116

[71] Rescigno G, Aratari C, Matteucci S, Parisi R, Gironi G, Schicchi N, D'Alfonso A, Cola V, Torracca L. Saphenous vein graft wrapping by nitinol mesh: A word of caution. Thoracic and Cardiovascular Surgeon. 2015;**63**:292-297. DOI: 10.1055/s-0034-1393705

[72] Taggart D, Ben Gal Y, Lees B, Patel N, Webb C, Rehman S, Desouza A, Yadav R, De Robertis F, Dalby M, Banning A, Channon K, Di Mario C, Orion E A randomized trial of external stenting for saphenous vein grafts in coronary artery bypass grafting. Annals of Thoracic Surgery. 2015;**99**:2039-2045. DOI: 10.1016/j.athoracsur.2015.01.060

[73] Verma S, Lovren F, Pan Y, Yanagawa B, Deb S, Karkhanis R, Quan A, Teoh H, Feder-Elituv R, Moussa F, Souza D, Fremes S. Pedicled no-touch saphenous vein graft harvest

limits vascular smooth muscle cell activation: The PATENT saphenous vein graft study. European Journal of Cardio-Thoracic Surgery 2014;**45**:717-725. DOI: 10.1093/ejcts/ezt560

[74] Souza D, Johansson B, Bojö L, Karlsson R, Geijer H, Filbey D, Bodin L, Arbeus M, Dashwood M. Harvesting the saphenous vein with surrounding tissue for CABG provides long-term graft patency comparable to the left internal thoracic artery: Results of a randomized longitudinal trial. Journal of Thoracic and Cardiovascular Surgery 2006;**132**:373-378. DOI: 10.1016/j.jtcvs.2006.04.002

[75] Samano N, Geijer H, Liden M, Fremes S, Bodin L, Souza D. The no-touch saphenous vein for coronary artery bypass grafting maintains a patency, after 16 years, comparable to the left internal thoracic artery: A randomized trial. Journal of Thoracic and Cardiovascular Surgery. 2015;**150**:880-888. DOI: 10.1016/j.jtcvs.2015.07.027

[76] Mills N, Everson C. Right gastroepiploic artery: A third arterial conduit for coronary artery bypass. Annals of Thoracic Surgery. 1989;**47**:706-711.

[77] Pym J, Brown P, Charrette E, Parker J, West R. Gastroepiploic-coronary anastomosis. A viable alternative bypass graft. Journal of Thoracic and Cardiovascular Surgery. 1987;**94**:256-259

[78] Suma H, Fukumoto H, Takeuchi A. Coronary artery bypass grafting by utilizing in situ right gastroepiploic artery: Basic study and clinical application. Annals of Thoracic Surgery. 1987;**44**:394-397.

[79] van Son J, Smedts F, Vincent J, van Lier H, Kubat K. Comparative anatomic studies of various arterial conduits for myocardial revascularization. Journal of Thoracic and Cardiovascular Surgery 1990;**99**:703-707.

[80] Suma H. The right gastroepiploic artery graft for coronary artery bypass grafting: A 30-year experience. Korean Journal of Thoracic and Cardiovascular Surgery. 2016;**49**:225-231. DOI: 10.5090/kjtcs.2016.49.4.225

[81] Suma H. Coronary artery bypass grafting in patients with calcified ascending aorta: Aortic no-touch technique. Annals of Thoracic Surgery 1989;**48**:728-730

[82] Suma H, Tanabe H, Takahashi A, Horii T, Isomura T, Hirose H, Amano A. Twenty years experience with the gastroepiploic artery graft for CABG. Circulation. 2007;**116**:I188-I191. DOI: 10.1161/CIRCULATIONAHA.106.678813

[83] Suzuki T, Asai T, Matsubayashi K, Kambara A, Kinoshita T, Takashima N, Hosoba S. In off-pump surgery, skeletonized gastroepiploic artery is superior to saphenous vein in patients with bilateral internal thoracic arterial grafts. Annals of Thoracic Surgery. 2011;**91**:1159-1164. DOI: 10.1016/j.athoracsur.2010.12.031

[84] Nishida H, Tomizawa Y, Endo M, Koyanagi H, Kasanuki H. Coronary artery bypass with only in situ bilateral internal thoracic arteries and right gastroepiploic artery. Circulation. 2001;**104**:I76-I80

[85] Hirose H, Amano A, Takanashi S, Takahashi A. Coronary artery bypass grafting using the gastroepiploic artery in 1000 patients. Annals of Thoracic Surgery 2002;**73**:1371-1379.

[86] Formica F, Ferro O, Greco P, Martino A, Gastaldi D, Paolini G. Long-term follow-up of total arterial myocardial revascularization using exclusively pedicle bilateral internal thoracic artery and right gastroepiploic artery. European Journal of Cardio-Thoracic Surgery. 2004;**26**:1141-1148. DOI: 10.1016/j.ejcts.2004.08.027

[87] Tavilla G, Kappetein A, Braun J, Gopie J, Tjien A, Dion R. Long-term follow-up of coronary artery bypass grafting in three-vessel disease using exclusively pedicled bilateral internal thoracic and right gastroepiploic arteries. Annals of Thoracic Surgery. 2004;**77**:794-799. DOI: 10.1016/S0003-4975(03)01659-X

Chapter 3

Left Main Coronary Artery Disease: Current Treatment Options

Omer Tanyeli

Additional information is available at the end of the chapter

http://dx.doi.org/10.5772/intechopen.71562

Abstract

Significant left main coronary artery disease is defined as a greater than 50% angiographic narrowing of the vessel. In general, there are three options for the treatment of LMCA disease which include optimal medical therapy, percutaneous revascularization, or surgical revascularization, either off-pump or on-pump. It is the highest-risk lesion subset of ischemic heart disease and until recent years, coronary artery bypass grafting was the major choice of treatment. Although there is a marked increase in use of percutaneous coronary intervention in left main disease, there are still some questions about its efficacy when compared with surgery. Although bypass surgery is the gold standard, current treatment guideline recommendations canalized the treatment of this potentially lethal disease into percutaneous interventions in selected patients who had low to intermediate anatomic complexity. Left main disease with low SYNTAX scores (≤22) can be treated either by bypass surgery or percutaneously, whereas SYNTAX score > 32 is an indication for only coronary artery bypass surgery. The heart team should always be in collaboration, give therapeutic options to patients and decide the best treatment strategy for the welfare of the patient.

Keywords: coronary artery disease, left main coronary artery disease, coronary artery bypass surgery, percutaneous intervention, PCI, CABG, SYNTAX score

1. Introduction

Despite its short length, the left main coronary artery (LMCA) is still one of the most challenging areas of disease for both cardiovascular surgeons and interventional cardiologists today. Significant LMCA disease is defined as a greater than 50% angiographic narrowing of the vessel. LMCA disease is the highest-risk lesion subset of ischemic heart disease and until recent years, coronary artery bypass grafting (CABG) was the major choice of treatment.

Although there is a marked increase in use of percutaneous coronary intervention (PCI) in LMCA disease, there are still some questions about its efficacy when compared with CABG operations. Starting from the traditional treatment options in LMCA disease, current treatment guideline recommendations canalized the treatment of this potentially lethal disease into PCI in selected patients who had low to intermediate anatomic complexity based on some scoring systems. Patient selection for both techniques is important and directly affects the clinical outcome. In this chapter, basic characteristics of the LMCA will be discussed with recommendations of treatment options under the highlights of recent studies and guidelines.

2. Importance of LMCA

The LMCA emerges from the aorta within the sinus of Valsalva through the ostia of the left aortic cusp. It passes between the pulmonary trunk and the left atrial appendage and just under the appendage; the artery divides into the left anterior descending (LAD) and the left circumflex coronary arteries (LCx). In one third of the patients, LMCA bifurcates into LAD, LCx and ramus intermedius branches [1]. The LMCA is responsible for supplying about 75% of the left ventricular (LV) cardiac mass in patients with right dominant type and 100% in the case of left dominant type, and as a result, severe LMCA disease will significantly reduce blood flow to a large portion of the myocardium and place the patient at high risk for life-threatening events, such as LV dysfunction and arrhythmias [2].

Significant LMCA disease is defined as greater than 50% angiographic narrowing of the artery and was shown to be present in about 4–6% of all patients who underwent coronary angiography [3]. Besides, patients with unprotected LMCA (ULMCA) disease treated medically have a 3-year mortality rate of about 50% [4].

The LMCA is anatomically divided into three portions: origin of LMCA from the aorta (ostium), mid portion and the distal portion. The LMCA is different from the other coronary arteries because it has relatively greater elastic tissue content; this feature explains the elastic recoil and its high restenosis rate, following balloon angioplasty procedures [5]. Since one-third of patients have trifurcated LMCA, this anatomical feature is important because in distal LMCA stenosis, PCI is much more difficult in trifurcated lesions than the bifurcated ones [6]. In 1% of the population, the LMCA is absent, and the LAD and LCx arteries originate directly from the aorta via separate ostia.

As with other coronary artery disease, the most common cause of LMCA disease is atherosclerosis. Non-atherosclerotic causes of LMCA lesions are rare. Other reasons may be either obstructive or nonobstructive. Since it is originated directly from the aorta, any disease affecting the ascending aorta can also cause LMCA obstruction such as aortic dissection, external compression resulting from aortic aneurysm or tumor, iatrogenic injury resulting from coronary interventions or vasospasm, irradiation, syphilitic aortitis, Takayasu's arteritis, rheumatoid arthritis, aortic valve disease including malposition of prosthesis, aneurismal dilatations such as Kawasaki disease and atherosclerotic aneurysms.

http://dx.doi.org/10.5772/intechopen.71562

There is a relationship between the length of LMCA and the LMCA segment that is diseased. In short LMCAs (<10 mm), the stenosis are more frequently localized at the ostium and then at the distal bifurcation (55 vs. 38%), in contrast to long LMCA that develops stenosis more frequently near the distal bifurcation compared to near the ostium (77 vs. 18%). The mid segment of LMS is rarely affected (5–7% of patients). Ostial LMCA stenoses are more common in women (44 vs. 20%) [7].

3. Diagnosis of LMCA disease

Most patients with LMCA disease are symptomatic. Since occlusion of this vessel compromises about 75% of blood flow to the LV, patients are at high risk of major cardiovascular events unless protected by a collateral flow. The diagnosis of LMCA disease is usually made by coronary angiography. The use of noninvasive imaging studies does not specifically distinguish LMCA from other types of coronary artery disease. Certain findings on exercise testing or, in patients with acute coronary syndromes on the electrocardiogram (ECG), are suggestive of LMCA disease. These include diffuse and severe ST-segment deviation or significant ventricular arrhythmias on ECG monitoring or hypotension during exercise [8].

Coronary angiography remains the gold standard diagnostic technique for the diagnosis of clinically important LMCA disease, although small but significant number of false-positive and false-negative results is present with inter-observer variabilities. In order to avoid precipitating myocardial ischaemia in patients with severe LMCA disease, operators try to limit the number of angiographic shots, as well as keep dye injections to a minimum: this may have an impact on diagnostic accuracy of less experienced operators. Ostial LMCA stenosis is not well shown angiographically; the diagnosis relies on detection of pressure damping on engagement of the ostia with the catheter tip and the absence of reflux of dye into the coronary sinus on injection. Detecting and quantifying stenosis of the LMCA and bifurcation rely on a normal segment for comparison: the severity of concentric stenoses of the entire LMCA may therefore be underestimated. Angiography is also poor at assessing lesion calcification. This is important firstly because where visual assessment is inaccurate, it is often because of the presence of calcification, and secondly because the presence of calcification is an important risk factor for dissection following PCI [9]. Coronary angiographic views of some patients with diagnosis of LMCA disease is shown in **Figure 1**.

In some cases, additional studies including intravascular ultrasound imaging (IVUS), fractional flow reserve (FFR) and coronary vasodilatory reserve (CVR) may be helpful for increasing diagnostic accuracy and decision-making.

IVUS is an intracoronary imaging modality that facilitates the anatomic visualization of the vessel lumen and characterizes plaques. It provides a 360° sagittal scan of the vessel from the lumen through the media to the vessel wall. It provides additional information such as minimal and maximal diameters, cross-sectional area and plaque area compared with coronary angiography alone [9]. IVUS detects calcification twice as often as angiography and is

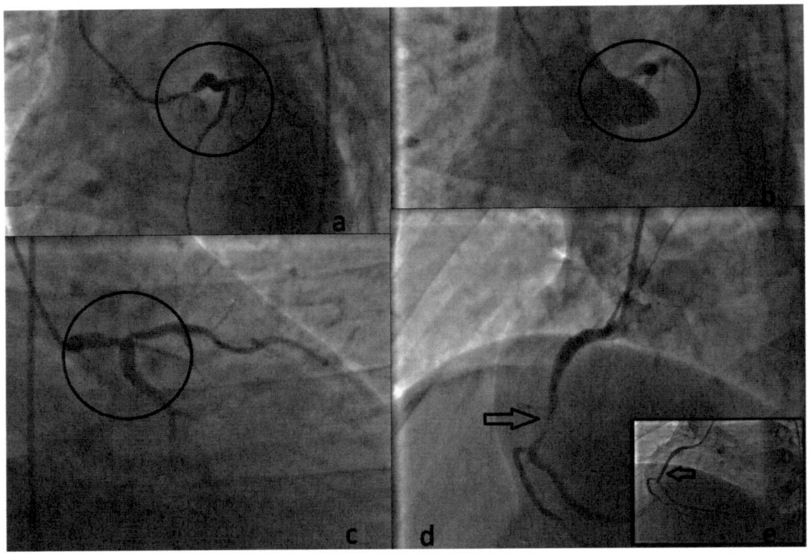

Figure 1. (a–b) Proximal LMCA stenosis at the level of aorto-ostial junction (in circles). (c–d) Acute MI patient with distal LMCA stenosis at the level of bifurcation and proximal part of LAD (in circle) and thrombosis of the RCA (arrow). (e) After thrombolytic infusion and balloon angioplasty flow in RCA is restored, patient is operated in elective conditions for left main disease.

more sensitive at detecting significant LMCA stenosis than angiography alone. IVUS may have a role in the assessment of high-risk patients and in deciding whether patients with angiographically indeterminate LMCA lesions should undergo PCI or surgery [10]. Since IVUS is an effective method to examine the coronary architecture and extent of atherosclerotic plaque with changes in vessel dimensions, it should be considered in angiographically borderline lesions as a complimentary method.

FFR is the ratio of distal coronary pressure to aortic pressure measured during maximal hyperemia which represents fraction of normal blood flow through a stenotic artery. The normal FFR for all vessels under all hemodynamic conditions, regardless of the status of the microcirculation, is 1.0. FFR values <0.75 are associated with abnormal stress tests [10]. FFR may have a role in deciding whether patients with angiographically mild or moderate LMCA disease should undergo revascularization: 56% of patients with FFR <0.75 in one study had significant LMCA stenoses [11].

CVR is the ratio of hyperemic to basal flow and reflects flow resistance through the epicardial artery and the corresponding myocardial bed. Unlike FFR, the value is affected by the coronary microcirculation and hemodynamic conditions. Although of use in the further assessment of angiographically indeterminate lesions, no studies have specifically addressed the use of this diagnostic adjunct in assessment of LMCA disease [10].

A LM pattern on exercise nuclear testing is characterized by perfusion defects in the LAD and LCx territories (i.e., reduced nuclear tracer uptake in the septal, anterior and lateral walls). It may also be associated with a picture of "balanced" ischemia where there is uniform diminution of tracer uptake with stress, often indicative of LM with three-vessel disease. This may be accompanied by transient ischemic dilation (TID), which is considered present when the image of the left ventricular cavity appears to be significantly greater after stress as compared with that at rest [12].

More recently cardiac CT and MRI have been shown to have a high correlation with angiography for the diagnosis of LM disease. This may be particularly useful in surveillance imaging after revascularization of the LM often performed after stenting [12]. Multislice computed tomography (MSCT), also called multidetector coronary angiography, has rapidly gained in popularity and applicability. MSCT has a good diagnostic accuracy for detecting more than 50% luminal stenosis with a sensitivity of 97% (CI: 94–98%) and specificity of 86% (CI: 78–90%) compared with quantitative conventional coronary angiography [13, 14].

Cardiovascular magnetic resonance imaging (CMRI) has some advantages and limitations compared with cardiac CT imaging. Advantages of CMRI include the absence of ionizing radiation and contrast media, as well as no requirement for heart rate control with b-blockers [12]. Detection of coronary lesions in heavily calcified coronary segments by CMRI can be more reliable than by cardiac CT [15].

There is a strong association between LMCA disease and carotid artery stenosis. Carotid artery disease is present in almost 40% of patients undergoing angiography for evaluation of angina, with significant left main stem disease, compared with just 5% with single-vessel disease [16]. The AHA guidelines recommend screening all patients undergoing bypass surgery for left main stem disease to identify carotid artery disease [17].

4. Preventive and medical therapies

There are three options for treating LMCA disease: optimal medical therapy, PCI, or surgical revascularization (CABG). All patients with LMCA disease should receive preventive therapies to decrease the risk of subsequent cardiovascular events. Preventive therapies include smoking cessation, exercise, lipid lowering therapy with stains, management of diabetes mellitus with proper oral antidiabetics or insulin and achievement of target blood pressure goals with suitable antihypertensive medications. In the 1970s and 1980s, three randomized controlled trials (the Veterans Affairs Cooperative Study [18], European Coronary Surgery Study [19], and CASS (Coronary Artery Surgery Study) [20]) established the survival benefit of CABG compared with contemporaneous medical therapy without revascularization in certain subjects with stable angina. They reported a survival rate of 80–88% for CABG and 63–68% for medical treatment only. Subsequently, a 1994 meta-analysis of 7 studies that randomized a total of 2649 patients to medical therapy for CABG showed that CABG offered a survival advantage over medical therapy for patients with LMCA disease or three-vessel coronary artery disease (CAD) [21]. The studies also established that CABG is more effective than medical therapy at relieving anginal symptoms.

5. Treatment of significant LMCA disease

In general, there are three options for the treatment of LMCA disease, which include optimal medical therapy, percutaneous revascularization, or surgical revascularization, either off-pump or on-pump. Hybrid procedures may also be applied according to patient's clinical status or clinician's choice for different scenarios.

As stated above, CABG offers a survival advantage over medical therapy for significant LMCA disease since medical therapy alone has been associated with poor outcomes. CABG surgery has been accepted as the standard revascularization method for LMCA disease for several decades. In the last decade, several randomized controlled trials have shown favorable results for PCI with drug-eluting stents (DES) compared with CABG. In this title of the chapter, scoring systems for decision making and treatment strategies for LMCA disease will be discussed, mainly focusing on the surgical treatment of LMCA disease.

Compared with the early days, contemporary bypass surgery has been greatly refined. Cardiopreservation techniques have improved and nearly all patients with LMCA disease receive an internal mammary artery (IMA) graft. In addition, patients undergoing surgery are more aggressively treated medically. The outcomes are excellent. When comparing the results of CABG with PCI, the coronary stents must perform at least as well as surgery in terms of outcomes [22].

A percutaneous approach for revascularization in LMCA disease has both attractive and undesirable features. Surgery needs a long recovery period with significant potential morbidities including postsurgical atrial fibrillation, pleural effusions, infections, delayed wound healing, anemia and depression which have negative effects on patient's quality of life. A percutaneous approach is clearly more palatable to patients than surgery. For the physician, LM stem is large and easily accessible for PCI techniques. However, especially for the patients with absent collateral vasculature, balloon inflation may lead to cardiovascular collapse with ischemia. Abrupt vessel closure or subsequent stent thrombosis involving the LM stem may be a fatal event. All of these factors must be taken into account and their effect clearly understood when comparing the two revascularization methods [22].

6. Scoring systems for decision-making in LMCA disease

The assessment of patients with LMCA disease both as a candidate for surgery or PCI is often a complex procedure and best achieved by the "Heart Team" approach. When one method of revascularization is preferred over the other for improved survival, this consideration takes precedence over improved symptoms. ACCF/AHA guideline suggests that a Heart Team approach to revascularization is recommended in patients with unprotected LM or complex CAD (Class I recommendation, Level of evidence; C) [17].

Several risk stratification scores, based on either angiographic or clinical parameters, have been developed to evaluate outcomes in patients with LMCA disease who undergo bypass surgery. Despite the use of various objective scoring systems derived from hundreds of thousands of patients, an experienced surgeon who spends time evaluating the coronary angiogram, taking a detailed history and examining the patient may provide the most accurate assessment of operative risk [22].

The Synergy between PCI with TAXUS and Cardiac Surgery (SYNTAX) score includes factors of coronary angiographic complexity rather than clinical factors. Although the limitations of using the SYNTAX score for certain revascularization recommendations are recognized, the SYNTAX score is a reasonable surrogate for the extent of CAD and its complexity and serves as important information that should be considered when making revascularization decisions. Recommendations that refer to SYNTAX scores use them as surrogates for the extent and complexity of CAD [17].

ACCF/AHA guideline suggests that calculation of the SYNTAX and STS (The Society of Thoracic Surgeons) scores is reasonable in patients with unprotected LM and complex CAD (Class IIa recommendation, level of evidence; B). Variables which contribute to the determination of the score include dominance of the coronary artery system, number of lesions, segment involved per lesions and presence of chronic total occlusions, trifurcation, bifurcation, aorto-ostial lesions, tortuosity, calcification, thrombi, long lesions and/or diffuse disease. By the highlights of these variables, a separate number is calculated for each lesion. Then, these values are summed up to generate the total SYNTAX score. An online tool for easy calculation of the score may be found online at http://www.syntaxscore.com. Some of the steps illustrating the scoring are shown in **Figure 2**.

SYNTAX trial is the largest, single published study to date, comparing the outcome of PCI vs. CABG in patients with 3-vessel coronary disease and LMCA disease [23]. The higher the score, the greater is the extent and the complexity of the disease. The SYNTAX trial stratified the entire randomized population (i.e., both patients with 3-vessel and patients with left main coronary artery disease) by tercile of SYNTAX score and found that the patients in the lowest tercile (score:0–22) fared just as well with PCI as surgery, whereas those in the highest tercile (score ≥ 33) clearly did better with surgery [22, 23]. Capodanno et al. applied the SYNTAX score to a registry of 819 patients undergoing LM PCI or surgery and found that the outcomes of patients with SYNTAX score ≥ 34 was better with surgery as compared with PCI but patients with SYNTAX score < 34 had similar outcomes with surgery or PCI in terms of 2-year mortality rates [24]. They concluded that a SYNTAX score threshold of 34 may usefully identify a cohort of patients with LMCA disease who benefit most from surgical revascularization in terms of mortality.

The SYNTAX study included a subset of 705 patients with LM stem disease and their 5-year outcomes have been published [25, 26]. For the overall group with LMCA disease, there was no significant difference in the rate of major adverse cardiac and cardiovascular events (MACCE), MI, or death at 5 years in patients treated with PCI compared with those treated with surgery [26]. The rate of stroke was lower in patients treated with PCI, and the rate of repeat revascularization was lower in patients treated with surgery. When the LM cohort was divided into two groups based on the SYNTAX score, striking differences between the

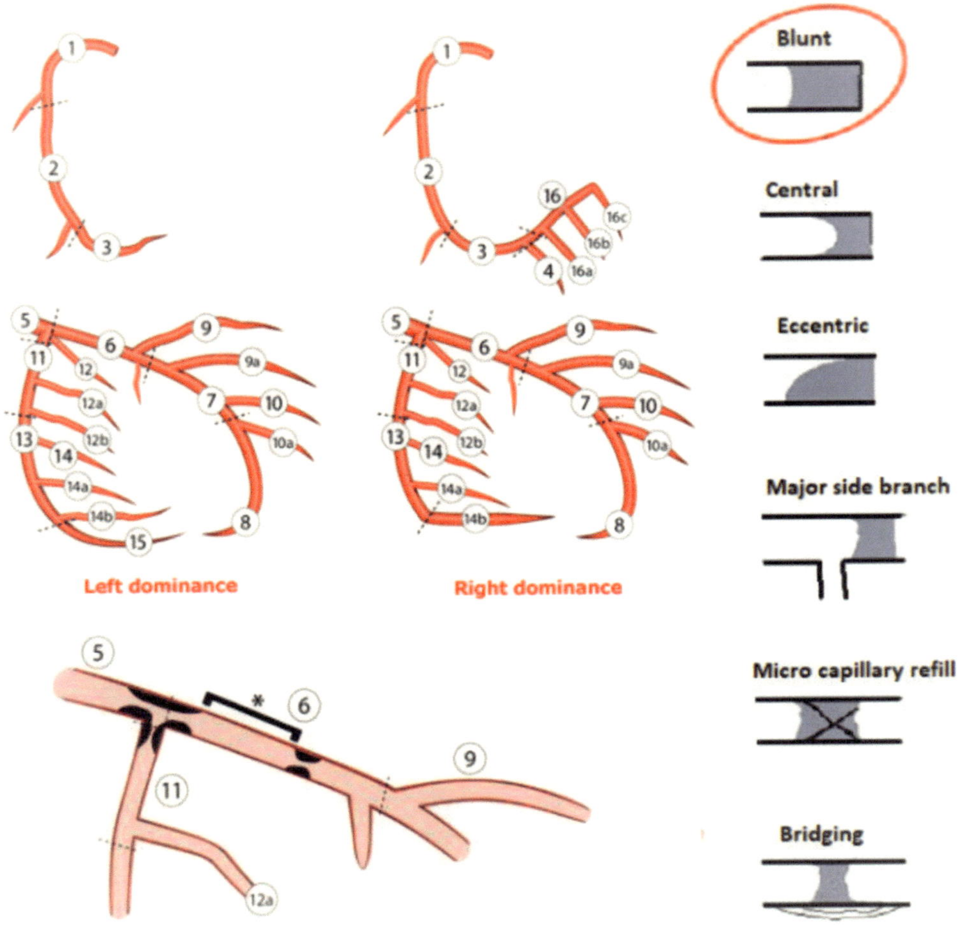

Figure 2. Some of the steps illustrating the SYNTAX scoring system; available online at: http://www.syntaxscore.com.

treatment strategies became apparent. For the high SYNTAX score group (≥33), the rate of MACCE was significantly greater in the PCI group compared with surgery. Although not statistically powered for mortality, the rate of death trended alarmingly higher in the PCI group. By contrast, for patients with scores <33, there was no difference in MACCE. Interestingly, in this group with low or intermediate scores, there was actually a lower mortality rate with PCI [22, 25, 26].

By-time, not only the anatomical assessment, but also the clinical status of the patients was added for better evaluation of the risk stratification, mainly on the SYNTAX score. The clinical SYNTAX score is a combination of age, creatinine and ejection fraction (ACEF) model and SYNTAX scores, and subsequent development of a logistic model has provided better risk assessment [27]. The SYNTAX II score is a combination of anatomical and clinical factors (age, creatinine clearance, LV function, gender, chronic obstructive pulmonary disease, and peripheral vascular disease) and predicts long-term mortality in patients with complex three-vessel

Recommendations according to extent of coronary artery disease	CABG		PCI	
	Class	Level of evidence	Class	Level of evidence
Left main disease with a SYNTAX score ≤ 22.	I	B	I	B
Left main disease with a SYNTAX score 23–32.	I	B	*IIa*	B
Left main disease with a SYNTAX score > 32.	I	B	*III*	B
Three vessel disease with a SYNTAX score ≤ 22.	I	A	I	B
Three vessel disease with a SYNTAX score 23–32.	I	A	*III*	B
Three vessel disease with a SYNTAX score > 32.	I	A	*III*	B

Table 1. ESC/EACTS recommendations for the type of revascularization in patients with left main coronary artery disease [30].

or LMCA disease [28]. It was found to be superior to the conventional SYNTAX score in guiding decision-making between CABG and PCI in the SYNTAX trial and subsequently validated in the drug-eluting stent for LMCA disease DELTA registry.

The STS score is a risk-prediction model, validated in patients undergoing cardiac surgery, with a specific model for CABG and combined CABG and valve surgery. It can be used to predict in-hospital or 30-day mortality and in-hospital morbidity [29]. ESC/EACTS guidelines on myocardial revascularization suggest STS score for CABG to assess short-term outcomes for CABG (Class IB recommendation) and SYNTAX score for both CABG and PCI to assess medium- to long-term (≥1 year) outcomes (Class IB recommendation) [30]. LMCA disease with low SYNTAX scores (≤22) should be treated either by CABG or PCI, whereas SYNTAX score > 32 is a contraindication for PCI. Recommendations of the ESC/EACTS guidelines for LMCA disease are summarized in **Table 1**.

7. Treatment of LMCA disease with PCI

Although surgery was and still is the main treatment option for unprotected LMCA disease, the emerging practice in PCI techniques and new materials has led to almost routine therapeutic option for a subset group of patients with LMCA disease. PCI for treatment of unprotected LMCA disease has passed through several phases. The early published experiences of balloon angioplasty for LMCA disease were associated with a high procedural mortality and poor long-term survival. In the 1980s, O'Keefe et al. reported 9.1% procedural mortality and 36% 3-year survival rate for 127 acute and elective cases with LMCA disease for coronary angioplasty [31]. In the following years, coronary stents improved the safety of PCI and also reduced the incidence of restenosis and abrupt vessel closure. As a result, these techniques were also used for a subset group of patients with LMCA disease. Initial experiences were performed with bare-metal stents and highly variable results were demonstrated according to studied patient population. Worse outcomes were published with cardiogenic shock and who were not surgical candidates, whereas god results were obtained in elective patients who were good surgical candidates. The bare-metal stent era was characterized by high restenosis and repeat revascularization rates, and restenosis of the LM stents resulted in sudden cardiac deaths [22].

After clinical use of drug-eluting stents, a reduction in restenosis rates renewed enthusiasm for PCI in LMCA disease. At first, different series reported better outcomes with drug-eluting stents for LMCA disease but their results were limited by selection bias regarding the patient characteristics and the anatomical features of LM stem [32]. For better understanding of the results, finally properly designed, large-scale randomized controlled trials comparing PCI with drug-eluting stents to CABG surgery emerged and they provided important answers to the question of PCI vs. CABG surgery for LMCA disease [22].

PCI for LMCA may exist with a broad spectrum of clinical scenarios. The LM stem may eventually be injured and closed as a complication of diagnostic cardiac catheterization. This iatrogenic injury might not be suitable for emergency operation and this patient may suddenly become a candidate for PCI. In a similar fashion, coronary flow of the patient in the cath lab for acute MI who has an occluded LM stem may rapidly be restored by PCI rather than surgery and this may be life-saving. Different preoperative risk assessment and scoring systems may demonstrate high operative risk for the patient, or the patient himself may simply refuse the operation, which automatically puts the patient in the PCI group. The most controversial group is the group of patients who are good surgical candidates and willing to be operated. Currently, surgery is considered the standard of care for this group. Many clinicians feel that PCI should not yet be offered to this group until the results of properly performed clinical trials comparing the outcomes of surgery vs. PCI are available and show that PCI outcomes are at least equal to those with surgery [22]. If left main PCI is being considered, it should not be performed immediately after coronary arteriography. The patient should hear opinions from a multidisciplinary team prior to deciding on a revascularization strategy. Exceptions to this principle include patients who are unstable and need immediate revascularization in the catheterization laboratory or those in whom CABG is not an option for any reason [8].

In a study designed by Erglis et al. comparing drug eluting stents and bare metal stents for the treatment of unprotected LMCA disease, 103 patients with stable angina were assigned to receive either paclitaxel-eluting stent or bare-metal stent. All interventions were IVUS guided and CB pre-treated before stenting was performed in all patients. All patients were scheduled for 6-month follow-up. Follow-up analysis showed binary restenosis in 11 (22%) bare-metal stent and in 3 (6%) paclitaxel-eluting stent patients ($p = 0.021$). The findings demonstrated that implantation of paclitaxel-eluting stents was superior to bare-metal stent in the large-diameter LM vessel at 6 months [33]. By the highlights of studies and improving stent technology, drug-eluting stents are preferred in general use for LMCA disease.

In the LMCA disease, the results for distal LM were worse when compared to ostial or midshaft lesions. Although long-term outcomes in patients with ostial/shaft unprotected LMCA lesions were favorable, outcomes in patients with bifurcation lesions treated with stenting of both the main and side branches appeared unacceptable [34]. The distal LMCA is the usual site of restenosis and the circumflex origin is especially vulnerable to restenosis.

In the ostial involvement, delineating the aorto-ostium by coronary angiography may be difficult and optimal stent decision may be tricky. The implantation of the stent for ostial LMS stenosis must be done with a small protrusion into the aorta to ensure adequate ostium coverage. The aorto-ostium may be very rigid due to calcium and has a tendency to recoil. In case of heavy calcification, rotational thrombectomy may help reducing calcium load, so that it helps balloon and stent expansion and prevents recoil. In most cases of ostial disease, IVUS proves very helpful to ensure coverage and proper stent expansion [22].

Distal LMS stenosis can be treated by a single-stent or by a two-stent strategy. The choice of the strategy is based on: plaque distribution, the angle between the two branches, the diameter of LAD and LCx and the presence of side branch stenosis [6]. Although the data are challenging, patients with distal LM stenosis treated with single-stent strategy have a TVR rate relatively low (<5%), nearly equivalent to patients with ostial or mid-shaft LM stenosis treated by the same strategy [35]. Provisional T-stenting is the most frequent used strategy for single-stent strategy. It consists of the deployment of a single stent from LMCA to the LAD or LCx, whichever has the highest diameter. T-stenting has an advantage that it allows placement of a second stent into the side branch if it is severely narrowed. In two-stent strategy, two stents are planned and deployed in one of several different ways (culotte method, double kissing crush, etc.) to treat both the main branch and the side branch. The lack of randomized data in this area makes it difficult to advocate one strategy over another.

In the "Intracoronary Stenting and Angiographic Results: Drug-eluting Stents for Unprotected LM Lesions" (ISAR-LM) randomized trial, comparing PCI with sirolimus-eluting stent vs. paclitaxel-eluting stent, no significant differences were reported in the composite outcome of death, MI, and TLR at 12-month follow-up. No difference was reported also in restenosis and 2-year LM-specific revascularization [36].

The best available data for long-term outcomes with stenting of LMCAD come from the EXCEL and NOBLE randomized trials. EXCEL trial assigned 1905 patients with LMCA disease of low or intermediate complexity (SYNTAX score ≤ 32) to either PCI with everolimus-eluting stents or CABG [37]. The primary endpoint, a composite of death from any cause, stroke, or MI at 3 years, occurred at a similar rate in both groups. There were no significant between-group differences in the three-year rates of the components of the primary endpoint. The secondary endpoint of death, stroke, or MI at 30 days occurred less often in patients in the PCI group due mainly to a lower rate of MI. The secondary endpoint of death, stroke, MI, or ischemia driven revascularization at 3 years occurred more often with PCI. PCI with everolimus-eluting stents was noninferior to CABG with respect to the rate of the composite endpoint of death, stroke, or myocardial infarction at 3 years.

The NOBLE trial randomly assigned 1201 patients (without ST-elevation MI) to complete revascularization with either PCI, using a biolimus-eluting stent, or CABG [38]. The primary endpoint of major adverse cardiac or cerebrovascular events (a composite of all-cause mortality, nonprocedural MI, any repeat coronary revascularization, and stroke) at 5 years occurred more often with PCI attributable mainly to more frequent revascularization in the PCI group and a higher rate of stroke, the latter of which is not consistent with all other trials. The findings of this study suggest that CABG might be better than PCI for treatment of LM stem CAD.

Sometimes, a patient with acute MI and demonstrated three-vessel disease with involvement of LMCA disease may benefit from emergency coronary angioplasty. If the responsible vessel for acute MI is the RCA and complicated with cardiogenic shock, direct PTCA for RCA may significantly reduce in-hospital mortality and the patient may become a surgical candidate for LMCA after evaluation of the mitral valve for ischemic mitral insufficiency for possible interventions in a more stable status.

Most of the LM PCI does not require hemodynamic support, but during PCI for LMCA disease, the operator should be ready for any hemodynamic compromise, slow or no reflow or other procedural complications and take necessary precautions. These precautions include the placement of intraaortic balloon pump (IABP) or sometimes the support of percutaneous LV assist devices in poor LV functions, such as the Impella. Patients more likely to need support include those with severe LV dysfunction, occlusion of the right coronary artery, a left dominant circulation, and patients in whom the PCI procedure is likely to be complex and difficult, thus increasing the ischemic time [22]. In general, careful attention to patient's baseline hemodynamic status before and during the procedure is necessary. Patient with instable hemodynamic status or those in whom even brief balloon inflations result in hemodynamic compromise may benefit from the support. As a member of the heart team, a cardiac surgeon should always be informed before the implementation of PCI for unprotected LMCA and the surgical team should be ready for any potential complications and eventually for emergency CABG.

Patients with a patent bypass graft to either the LAD or LCx, who are considered to be "protected," may require LM intervention because of recurrent ischemia. Protected lesions are anatomically similar to those that are not previously bypassed. However, their physiology during treatment and the consequences of abrupt closure and restenosis are much more forgiving because of continued flow to the protected territory [8].

8. Surgical treatment of LMCA disease

LMCA disease is an important independent risk factor for increased mortality and morbidity at all stages of diagnosis and treatment of CAD. For several decades, CABG was regarded as the standard of care for significant LMCA disease in patients eligible for surgery. More recently, PCI has emerged as a possible alternative method of treatment for revascularization in specifically selected, especially low risk group of patients, except for the life-saving emergency high-risk groups. Besides patient characteristics, lesion location is an important factor for the determination of treatment of choice as well as operator's experience and technical considerations. Stenting of distal stem or bifurcation lesions is technically challenging and most of the patients are presented with three-vessel disease which makes them good surgical candidates. Although the improvement in stent technology and increased experience of PCI techniques by the operators sometimes make the surgery questionable, surgery is still the "gold standard" for treatment of LMCA disease [24]. The outcomes of patients with SYNTAX score ≥ 34 was better with surgery as compared with PCI CABG surgery, which improves survival in patients with significant LMCA disease, three-vessel (and possibly two-vessel) disease, or reduced ventricular function, and prolongs and improves the quality of life in patients with LM equivalent disease (proximal LAD and proximal LCx), but does not protects them from the risk of subsequent MI. In this section, patient selection and CABG methods, as well as technical considerations, will be discussed for surgical treatment of LMCA disease. Indications of surgery for LMCA disease in ACCF/AHA guideline is summarized in **Table 2.**

By far, the most common known etiology of LMCA disease is atherosclerosis. Non-atherosclerotic causes of LMCA lesions are rare. Since atherosclerosis is a generalized disease affecting the whole arterial system in the body, its association should always be kept in mind such as carotid artery disease, cerebrovascular disease and peripheral artery disease as well as porcelain aorta which make the surgical procedure more challenging.

The incidence of sudden death in patients with critical LMCA disease means that these patients should never be thought as patients in the waiting list for elective surgery. Emergency CABG is recommended as Class I indication for patients with life-threatening ventricular arrhythmias, which is believed to be ischemic in origin, in the presence of ≥50 LMCA stenosis [17]. In a study by Maziak et al. [39], patients in the waiting list for CABG operations were evaluated. In this study, 281 patients over 2145 had critical (≥50%) LM stenosis. The average time from angiography to operation was shorter in patients with LMCA disease and the presence of LMCA disease did not influence operative mortality, the incidence of low cardiac output syndrome or the incidence of perioperative MI. To examine the effect of waiting time on outcomes, patients with LMS were divided into early (operation 10 days or less after angiography) and late revascularization groups (more than 10 days). Operative mortality, low output syndrome, and myocardial infarction were similar in the early and late groups. Patients in the early group were more likely to have NYHA functional Class IV symptoms, unstable angina, or a recent preoperative myocardial infarction. He concluded that carefully selected patients with significant LMS can safely wait for operation. But, it should be kept in mind that patients with severe symptoms and recently preoperative MI should be allocated for early surgical intervention.

The "Heart Team," made up of clinical or noninvasive cardiologists, cardiac surgeons and interventional cardiologists, provides a balanced, multidisciplinary decision-making process. Formulation of the best possible revascularization approaches, also taking into consideration the social and cultural context, will often require interaction between these branches. Patients may need help in making decisions about their treatment and the most valuable advice will probably be provided to them by the Heart Team [40].

Class I indications	• *CABG in Patients With Acute MI:* Emergency CABG is recommended in patients with life-threatening ventricular arrhythmias (believed to be ischemic in origin) in the presence of LM stenosis ≥50% and/or 3-vessel CAD *(LoE: C)* • *Life-Threatening Ventricular Arrhythmias:* CABG is recommended in patients with resuscitated sudden cardiac death or sustained ventricular tachycardia thought to be caused by significant CAD (>50% stenosis of LMCA and/or >70% stenosis of 1, 2, or all 3 epicardial coronary arteries) and resultant myocardial ischemia *(LoE: B)* • *CABG in Association With Other Cardiac Procedures:* CABG is recommended in patients undergoing noncoronary cardiac surgery ≥50% luminal diameter narrowing of the LMCA or ≥70% luminal diameter narrowing of other major coronary arteries *(LoE: C)* • *Heart Team Approach to Revascularization Decisions*: A Heart Team approach to revascularization is recommended in patients with unprotected LM or complex CAD *(LoE: C)* • *Left Main CAD Revascularization:* CABG to improve survival is recommended for patients with significant (>50% diameter stenosis) left main coronary artery stenosis *(LoE: B)*
Class IIa indications	• Calculation of the STS and SYNTAX scores is reasonable in patients with unprotected LM and complex CAD *(LoE: B)* • *Left Main CAD Revascularization:* 1. PCI to improve survival is reasonable as an alternative to CABG in selected stable patients with significant (>50% diameter stenosis) unprotected LMCAD with: (1) anatomic conditions associated with a low risk of PCI procedural complications and a high likelihood of good long-term outcome (e.g., a low SYNTAX score [<22], ostial or trunk left main CAD); and (2) clinical characteristics that predict a significantly increased risk of adverse surgical outcomes (e.g., STS-predicted risk of operative mortality >5%) *(LoE: B)* 2. PCI to improve survival is reasonable in patients with UA/NSTEMI when an unprotected LMCA is the culprit lesion and the patient is not a candidate for CABG *(LoE: B)* 3. PCI to improve survival is reasonable in patients with acute STEMI when an unprotected LMCA is the culprit lesion, distal coronary flow is <TIMI grade 3, and PCI can be performed more rapidly and safely than CABG *(LoE: C)* • Carotid artery duplex scanning is reasonable in selected patients who are considered to have high-risk features (i.e., age > 65 years, LMC stenosis, PAD, history of cerebrovascular disease (transient ischemic attack (TIA), stroke, etc.), hypertension, smoking, and diabetes mellitus) *(LoE: C)* • In the absence of severe, symptomatic aorto-iliac occlusive disease or PAD, the insertion of an IAB is reasonable to reduce mortality rate in CABG patients who are considered to be at high risk (e.g., those who are undergoing reoperation or have LVEF <30% or LMCAD) *(LoE: B)*
Class IIb indications	• *Left Main CAD Revascularization:* PCI to improve survival may be reasonable as an alternative to CABG in selected stable patients with significant (>50% diameter stenosis) unprotected LMCAD with: (1) anatomic conditions associated with a low to intermediate risk of PCI procedural complications and an intermediate to high likelihood of good long-term outcome (e.g., low–intermediate SYNTAX score of <33, bifurcation LMCAD); and (2) clinical characteristics that predict an increased risk of adverse surgical outcomes (e.g., moderate–severe chronic obstructive pulmonary disease, disability from previous stroke, or previous cardiac surgery; STS-predicted risk of operative mortality >2%) *(LoE: B)* • CABG to improve survival rate may be reasonable in patients with end-stage renal disease undergoing CABG for LMCA stenosis of ≥50% *(LoE: C)*

Class III indications (HARM)	• PCI to improve survival should not be performed in stable patients with significant (>50% diameter stenosis) unprotected LMCAD who have unfavorable anatomy for PCI and who are good candidates for CABG *(LoE: B)*

Abbreviations: CABG: coronary artery bypass graft; CAD: coronary artery disease; IAB: intraaortic balon; LM: left main; LMCAD; left main coronary artery disease; LoE: level of evidence; LVEF: left ventricle ejection fraction; NSTEMI: non-ST elevation myocardial infarction; PAD: peripheral artery disease; PCI: percutaneous coronary revascularization; UA; unstable angina.

Table 2. ACCF/AHA guideline recommendations for left main coronary artery bypass graft surgery [17].

The hospital mortality rate for CABG surgery is approximately 1% in low-risk patients, with fewer than 3% of patients suffering perioperative myocardial infarction. The most consistent predictors of mortality after CABG are urgency of operation, age, prior cardiac surgery, female gender, low LV ejection fraction, degree of LM stenosis, and number of vessels with significant stenoses. The most common mode of early death after CABG is acute cardiac failure leading to low output or arrhythmias, owing to myocardial necrosis (often with features of reperfusion), postischemic dysfunction of viable myocardium, or a metabolic cause, such as hypokalemia. As in cardiac surgery, in general, the risk of perioperative MI increases with the degree of cardiomegaly, and in patients who have had preoperative infarction [41].

8.1. Myocardial protection for surgery in LMCA disease

The objective of any type of myocardial management during cardiac surgery should target on decreasing injury to the myocardium by combination of hypothermia, electromechanical arrest, washout, oxygen and other substrate enhancement and buffering. There is no one specific method that ideally describes the myocardial protection as in the LMCA disease. It depends on surgeon's preferences, surgical technique, and surgeon's desire for complete bloodless area during the operation, sequence and timing of proximal anastomoses and costs. The optimum strategy for myocardial protection in severe LMCA disease remains unclear not only because of different regimens, but also the advanced stenosis of the LM stem resulting in uneven distribution of the preferred cardioplegic solution, slow diastolic arrest and delayed functional recovery due to pre- and perioperative functional status of the heart in critical LM stenosis and recent MI.

The myocardial protection is achieved by either antegrade blood cardioplegia through the ascending aorta via right and left coronary ostia in the absence of severe aortic regurgitation or retrograde blood cardioplegia by a special cannula inserted into the coronary sinus through the right atrium. Severe obstructive manifestations of CAD are perhaps the best examples for the superiority of retrograde cardioplegia. These include LM lesions and acute coronary syndromes. In this specific concern of LMCA disease, the cardioplegia distribution is not even because of the proximal stenosis and may cause impaired myocardial protection. Although retrograde cardioplegia results in better distribution, myocardial cooling and more complete functional recovery of myocardium distal to coronary artery stenoses, the presence of veno-venous shunts and thebesian channels means that distribution of retrograde cardioplegia may not effectively protect the right ventricle and posterior septum [42]. A combined approach may be a better alternative for myocardial protection where antegrade blood cardioplegia and maintained with continuous retrograde blood cardioplegia has been shown to result in reduced postoperative serum troponin I levels and rates of atrial fibrillation, compared with approaches using solely antegrade cardioplegia in patients with significant LMCA disease [43]. Patients with LMCA disease also have high incidences of involvement of RCA occlusion; so, not only the left coronary system, but also the right coronary system is impaired during antegrade cardioplegia route.

A conscious decision to use both the antegrade and retrograde routes of cardioplegia routinely, delivered in either an alternating sequential fashion or simultaneously, has evolved in the practice of some institutions. In our daily practice, we use combined antegrade and retrograde cardioplegia technique. In lack of severe aortic insufficiency, half or two-thirds of the dose is given through the antegrade perfusion cannula and the remaining solution is given through the retrograde cannula. After performing the first distal anastomosis by saphenous graft to the LCx system (mainly the best obtuse marginal artery branch), we do not wait for completion of time and perfuse the LCx from directly through the anastomosed saphenous vein graft, if the stenosis of LMCA disease is severe (**Figure 3**). In the absence of LAD stenosis, direct perfusion of LCx also allows perfusion of LAD in retrograde fashion.

Sometimes slow continuous retrograde perfusion may also be applied for better protection. Our goal is primarily good protection of the heart with as short cross-clamp time as possible. After completion of LIMA-LAD anastomosis, hot-shot with warm blood cardioplegia is given and usually the proximal anastomoses of the saphenous vein grafts to the ascending aorta is performed after the heart began to beat by the aid of side-clamp. If the aorta is severely calcified, single-clamp strategy may be used. Also, for better recovery of the heart, we also go on perfusing the heart by a line derived from the arterial cannula inserted into each saphenous vein grafts during proximal anastomosis stage.

Other preoperative prophylactic or postoperative insertion of the IABP is sometimes advisable. In addition to its use in MI with low cardiac output or shock, preoperative insertion is often helpful in unstable angina, LM disease with ongoing ischemia, and ischemia leading to ventricular arrhythmias. In the era of more complex arterial revascularization for ischemic heart disease, IABP support is helpful intraoperatively for pre-bypass support of patients with low ejection fraction [44]. When an IABP is used, it is important to understand that it is not the final therapy in terms of mechanical support for the failing heart. If the shock state persists, as evidenced by a depressed cardiac index, then some form of direct mechanical support must be implemented so as to restore adequate end-organ perfusion. Failure to adequately treat a patient in cardiogenic shock will most assuredly result in the patient's demise [41].

8.2. Type of surgery

Since the first CABG was performed in the late 1960s, the standard surgical approach has included the use of cardiac arrest coupled with CPB, optimizing the conditions for construction of

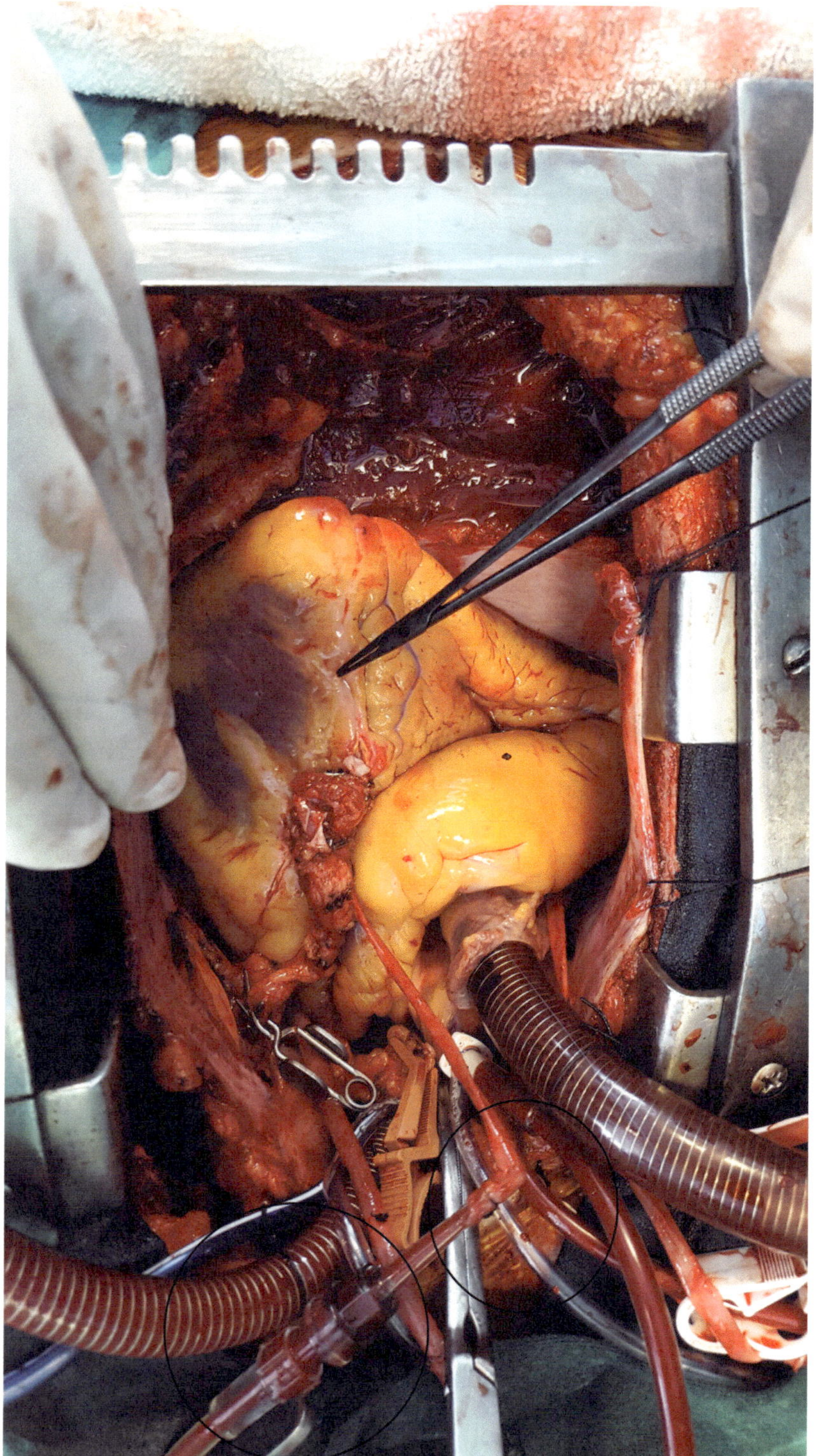

Figure 3. During on-pump bypass surgery, anastomosed saphenous vein grafts are perfused before LIMA-LAD anastomosis for better myocardial protection in left main coronary artery disease (in circle).

vascular anastomoses to all diseased coronary arteries without cardiac motion or hemodynamic compromise. Such on-pump CABG has become the gold standard and is performed in about 80% of subjects undergoing the procedure [17]. Despite the excellent results that have been achieved, the use of CPB and the associated manipulation of the ascending aorta are linked with certain perioperative complications, including myonecrosis during aortic occlusion, cerebrovascular accidents, generalized neurocognitive dysfunction, renal dysfunction, and systemic inflammatory response syndrome. To avoid these potential complications, off-pump surgical technique was developed by the aid of special cardiac stabilizing devices. This technique is also helpful in avoidance of touching the aorta which may be heavily calcified. In 2005, an AHA Scientific statement comparing the two techniques concluded that both procedures usually result in excellent outcomes and that neither technique should be considered superior to the other [45].

The LMCAD is known to be an important poor prognostic factor related to morbidity and mortality at various stages of CAD. In the past, LMCAD was accepted as a relative contraindication for off-pump CABG because of the hemodynamic compromise of the patient by changing the position of the heart. With evolving experience, some centers began to use off-pump technique in their routine daily practice and emerging number of reports in the literature have proven this method as a safe alternative to CPB. In a review article searching for studies comparing the results of on-pump CABG and off-pump CABG in patients with LMCAD, the outcomes, concerns and controversies were evaluated [46]. The majority of the studies identified showed favorable or equal outcomes of OFP when compared to conventional approach. All of the studies, apart from two, which showed lower incidence of postoperative deaths, demonstrated equal mortality rates. Stroke rates were found less in three studies. Less blood transfusions, inotropic use and length of study has been also demonstrated. The main concerns of off-pump surgery were hemodynamic instability and less complete revascularization. Main controversies were same or favorable outcomes, despite lower number of grafts with off-pump surgery, and less stroke rates, despite manipulation of aorta with side-clamping. Despite these concerns and controversies off-pump surgery has been proven to be feasible and safe as demonstrated by results from numerous studies.

Patients who have had recent MI with impaired LV and patients with dilated ventricles may not be ideal candidates for off-pump bypass procedures. Similarly, in patients with more than mild mitral insufficiency, grafting the branches of the LCx coronary artery may cause hemodynamic instability during the procedure. In such cases, surgery may be best managed by performing the revascularization procedure on the beating heart with cardiopulmonary support. The aorta is not clamped and cardioplegia is not administered. In such conditions, the heart is kept empty, providing optimal myocardial protection and hemodynamic stability (**Figure 4**).

Anesthetic management is very important during off-pump surgery. The key to avoiding conversion to emergency CPB should be proactive by preventing hypotension and low cardiac output. Intravascular volumes should be replenished before positioning the heart. The most common reason for hypotension is venous return problems. To prevent this, Trendelenburg position with turning the patient right-side may be helpful. The most important part for

http://dx.doi.org/10.5772/intechopen.71562

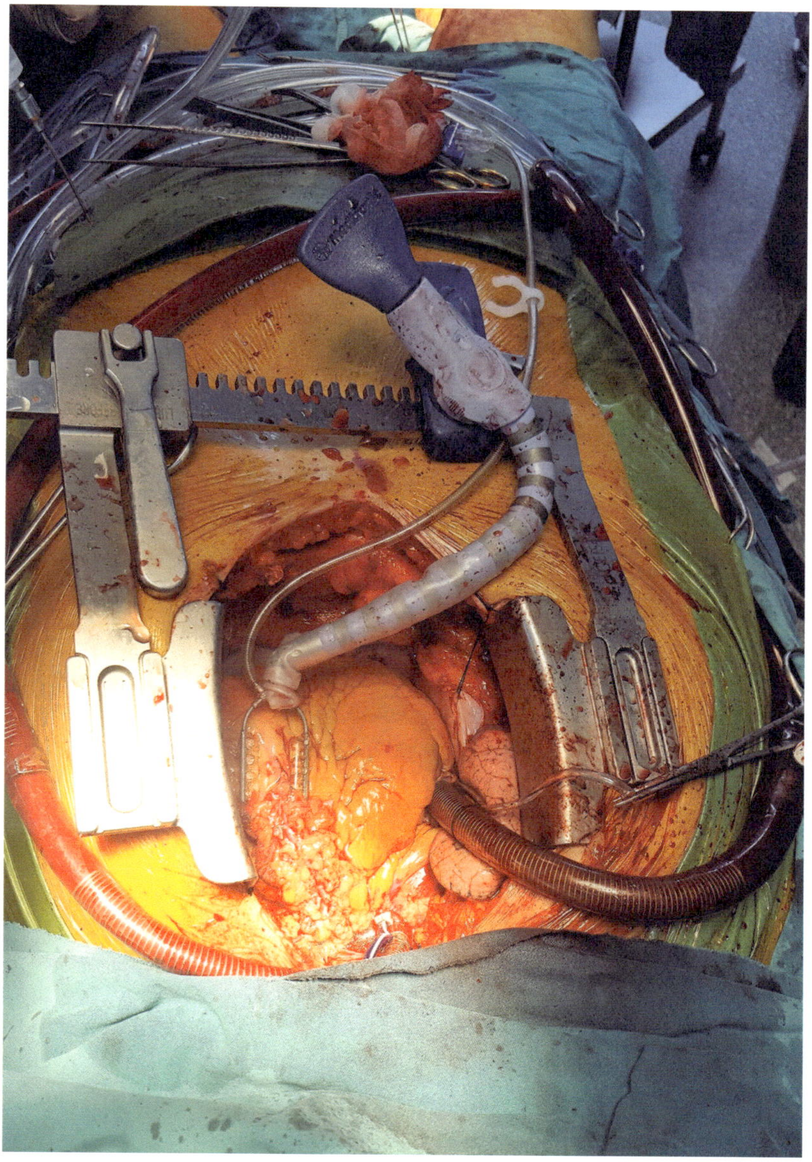

Figure 4. Cardiopulmonary bypass-assisted beating heart surgery. Note that the aorta is not clamped and cardioplegia is not administered. In such conditions, the heart is kept empty, providing optimal myocardial protection and hemodynamic stability.

positioning the heart is placement of the pericardial sutures. If the target vessel is on the left side, right side pericardial sutures should be left free and the deep pericardial sutures and the left pericardial sutures should be tightened. Generally, lifting the heart to a vertical position is relatively well tolerated. After carefully defining the target vessel, stabilizer device (e.g., Octopus System, Medtronic Inc. Minneapolis, MN) and their pads should be placed around the vessel at diastolic phase and be fixed. After the arteriotomy, placement of intra-arterial shunt provides myocardial blood flow continuity, minimizes distal bed ischemia and helps in correct suturing. During beating heart surgery, the operative field may become dirty because of bleeding; in that case silastic tape traction from proximal and distal portion of the arteriotomy may stop bleeding and help for a bloodless area. Carbondioxide mist blower is also helpful for clear view of the operating field.

Usually anterior and the most critic vessel should be anastomosed first. In LMCA disease, after preparation of the left internal mammarian artery (LIMA), direct anastomosis to LAD provides blood flow to LV. LAD artery is usually grafted at distal one-third to one-half where the artery normally emerges from the intramyocardial location if suitable. Other LCx obtuse marginal branches can be accessed with the heart in vertical position and rotated to the right. Use of apical suction devices may help positioning the heart. In LMCA disease, positioning of the heart may cause hemodynamic instability, especially after acute MI. After LAD anastomosis, if the hemodynamic instability persists, the patient may be a candidate for hybrid approach for future PCI. The goal of the surgery should be complete revascularization in normal conditions; but any unnecessary attempts to provide complete revascularization which threatens his life should be avoided.

8.3. Conduit selection

The effectiveness of CABG in relieving symptoms and prolonging life is directly related to graft patency. Because arterial and venous grafts have different patency rates and modes of failure, conduit selection is important in determining the long-term efficacy of CABG. The LIMA is the conduit of choice for revascularization of LAD distal to the LMCA lesion. LIMA should be used to bypass the LAD artery when bypass of the LAD artery is indicated (Class I recommendation for ACCF/AHA guideline for CABG surgery) [17].Since the atherosclerosis is an active event, anastomosis should be performed to the best distal area. LIMA provides superior short- and long-term patency and clinical outcomes to alternative conduits. Unlike saphenous vein grafts, IMA's are usually >90% patent after 10 years. They are resistant to atherosclerosis and release prostacyclin and nitric oxide, thereby causing vasodilation and inhibiting platelet function, by their endothelium studies suggesting an improved survival rate in patients undergoing CABG, when the LIMA is used rather than saphenous vein grafts to LAD. This survival benefit is independent of the patient's sex, age, extent of CAD, and LV systolic function [47]. Apart from improving survival rate, LIMA grafting of the LAD artery reduces the incidence of late MI, hospitalization for cardiac events, need for reoperation and recurrence of angina [48].

Although arterial conduits such as the radial artery have been shown to offer superior long-term patency to saphenous vein grafts, the risk of arterial graft spasm in the immediate postoperative period has discouraged some surgeons from total arterial revascularization of LMCA lesions [9]. Tatoulis et al. who analyzed 8420 patients, including 849 with significant LMCA disease, did not report adverse sequelae attributable to graft spasm in patients with LMCA disease who underwent total arterial grafting [49]. Patients should be informed before radial artery harvesting. Usually, the radial artery is harvested from the non-dominant arm of the patient. We routinely perform Doppler ultrasonography for evaluation of radial artery. The radial artery diameter >2 mm is usually suitable for a good quality conduit.

Dominance of the ulnar artery in hand should also be evaluated by modified Allen test [50]. Radial artery graft patency is best when used to graft a left-sided coronary artery with >70% stenosis and worst when it is used to bypass the right coronary artery with a stenosis of only moderate severity [51]. In technical aspects, we use radial artery grafts for >90% lesions and, during harvest, we use ultrasonic/harmonic scissors to avoid heat trauma to the vessel. After harvesting the graft, all the fasciae over the radial artery is also cleared longitudinally to prevent vasospasm (**Figure 5**). This maneuver also helps us making a better bleeding control from the side branches and provides better vessel diameter. Topical papaverine is also a good option for prevention of vasospasm.

Combination of LIMA, right IMA and radial artery may be used for full arterial revascularization processes. Some centers also prefer gastroepiploic artery either in case of inappropriate LIMA or in combination with LIMA and RIMA for full arterial revascularization concept (**Figure 6**).

Besides these arterial grafts, reversed saphenous vein grafts are commonly used in patients undergoing CABG surgery. Their disadvantage is a declining patency with time: about 10–25% of saphenous vein grafts occlude within 1 year of CABG [52]. An additional 1–2% occlude each year during the 1–5 years after surgery; and 4–5% occlude each year between 6 and 10 years postoperatively. Therefore, 10 years after CABG, 50–60% of saphenous vein grafts are patent, only half of which have no angiographic evidence of atherosclerosis [53].

Patient's age, stenosis degree of the affected coronary artery and hemodynamic status of the patient are important factors for overall graft selection. If possible, all patients with LMCA

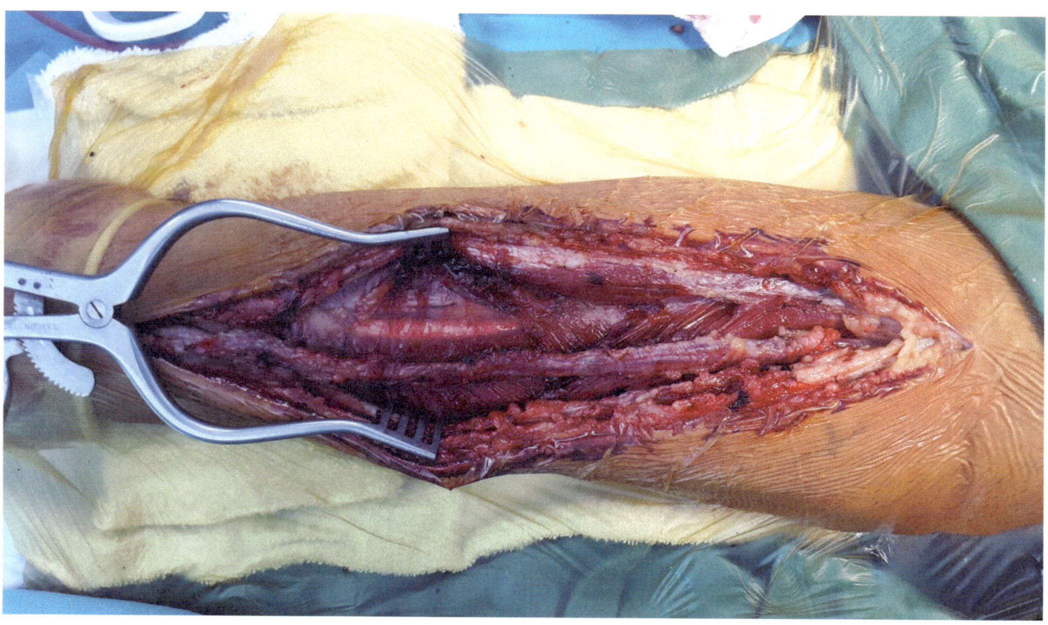

Figure 5. Radial artery harvesting with the fascia over the artery opened longitudinally to prevent vasospasm.

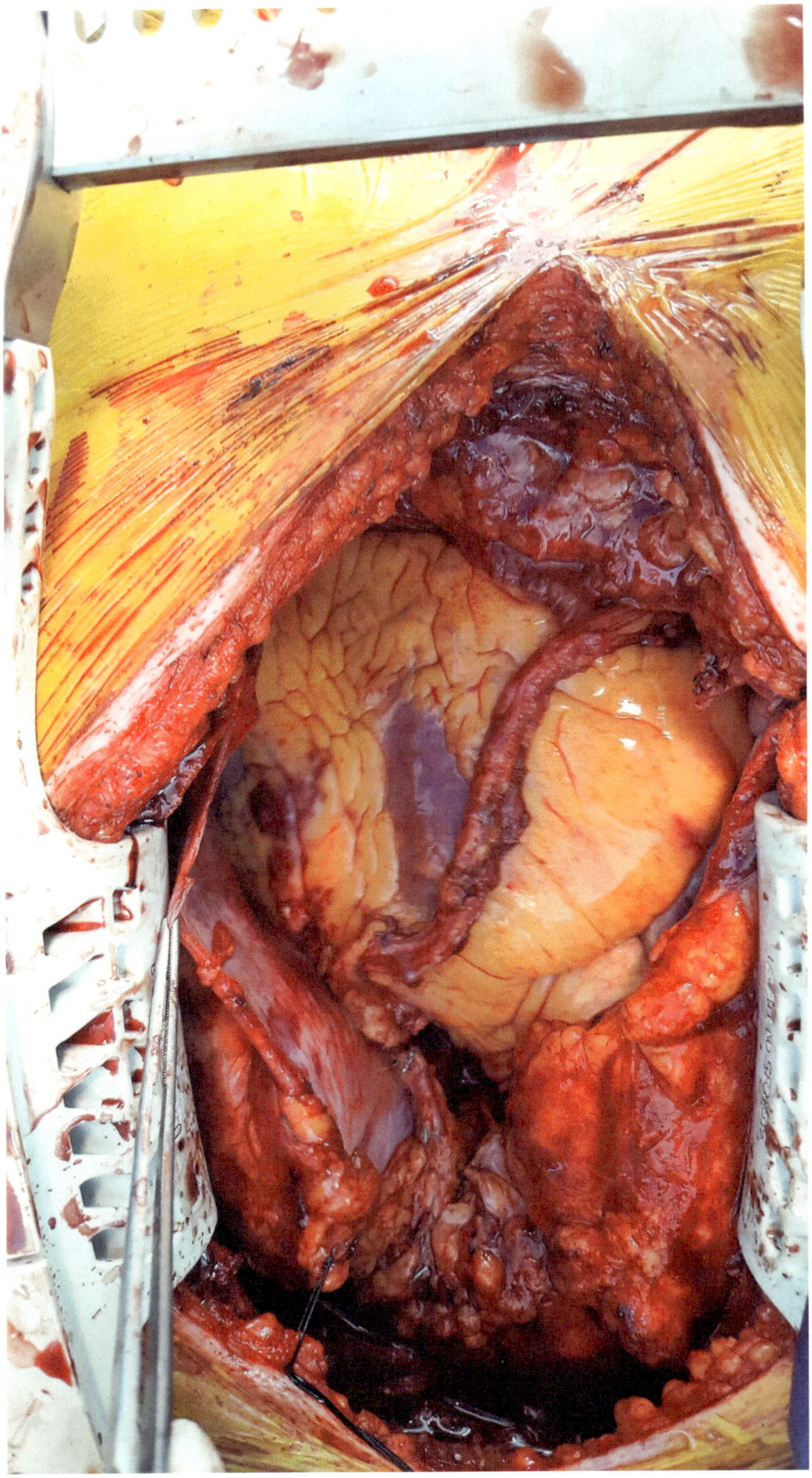

Figure 6. Arterial-only revascularization with LIMA-OM2 and RIMA-LAD anastomoses.

disease who are candidates for surgery deserve LIMA-LAD anastomosis either with on-pump or off-pump CABG surgery. Any surgeon should always target on full revascularization, but PCI should also be kept in mind. The heart team should also be in contact with LMCA patients not only before the operation, but also after the operation for future interventions or medical treatment plan.

9. Conclusion

LMCA disease is still one of the most challenging areas of disease for both cardiovascular surgeons and interventional cardiologists today. CABG offers a survival advantage over medical therapy for significant LMCA disease since medical therapy alone has been associated with poor outcomes. CABG surgery has been accepted as the standard revascularization method for LMCA disease for several decades. In the last decade, several randomized controlled trials have shown favorable results for PCI, and the emerging practice in PCI techniques and new materials has led to almost routine therapeutic option for a subset group of patients with LMCA disease. LMCA disease with low SYNTAX scores (≤22) can be treated either by CABG or PCI, whereas SYNTAX score > 32 is an indication for only CABG. The heart team should always be in collaboration, give therapeutic options to patients and decide the best treatment strategy for the welfare of the patient.

Author details

Omer Tanyeli

Address all correspondence to: otanyeli@gmail.com

Department of Cardiovascular Surgery, Meram Medicine Faculty, Necmettin Erbakan University, Konya, Turkey

References

[1] Park SJ, Park DW. Percutaneous coronary intervention with stent implantation versus coronary artery bypass surgery for treatment of left main coronary artery disease: Is it time to change guidelines? Circulation. Cardiovascular Interventions. 2009;**2**:59-68. DOI: 10.1161/CIRCINTERVENTIONS.108.831701

[2] Kalbfleisch H, Hort W. Quantitative study on the size of coronary artery supplying areas postmortem. American Heart Journal. 1977;**94**:183-188

[3] Ragosta M, Dee S, Sarembock IJ, Lipson LC, Gimple LW, Powers ER. Prevalance of unfavorable angiographic characteristics for percutaneous intervention in patients with unprotected left main coronary artery disease. Catheterization and Cardiovascular Interventions. 2006;**68**:357. DOI: 10.1002/ccd.20709

[4] Taylor H, Deumite N, Chaitman B, Davis K, Killip J, Rogers W. Asymptomatic left main coronary artery disease in the coronary artery surgery study (CASS) registry. Circulation. 1989;**79**:1171-1179. DOI: 10.1161/01.CIR.79.6.1171

[5] Macaya C, Alfonso F, Iniguez A, Goicolea J, Hernandez R, Zarco P. Stenting for elastic recoil during coronary angioplasty of the left main coronary artery. American Journal of CardiologyAmJ Cardiol. 1992;**70**:105-107

[6] Predescu LM, Zarma L, Platon P, Postu M, Bucsa A, Croitoru M, et al. Current treatment of left main coronary artery disease. Cor et Vasa. 2016;**58**:e328-e339

[7] Maehara A, Mintz GS, Castagna MT, Pichard AD, Satler LF, Waksman R, et al. Intravascular ultrasound assessment of stenosis location and morphology in the left main coronary artery in relation to anatomic left main length. American Journal of Cardiology. 2001;**88**:1-4. DOI: 10.1016/S0002-9149(01)01575-2

[8] Cutlip D, Aldea GS, Saperia GM. Management of Left Main Coronary Artery Disease. [Internet] Available from: http://www.uptodate.com/contents/management-of-left-main-coronary-artery-disease [Accessed Jul 10, 2017]

[9] Chikwe J, Kim M, Goldstone AB, Fallahi A, Athanasiou T. Current diagnosis and management of left main coronary disease. European Journal of Cardio-Thoracic Surgery. 2010;**38**:420-430. DOI: 10.1016/j.ejcts.2010.03.003

[10] Mintz GS, Popma JJ, Pichard AD, Kent KM, Satler LF, Chuang YC, et al. Patterns of calcification in coronary artery disease. A statistical analysis of intravascular ultrasound and coronary angiography in 1155 lesions. Circulation. 1995;**91**:1959-1965. DOI: 10.1161/01.CIR.91.7.1959

[11] Bech GJ, Droste H, Pijls NH, De Bruyne B, Bonnier JJ, Michels HR, et al. Value of fractional flow reserve in making decisions about bypass surgery for equivocal left main coronary artery disease. Heart. 2001;**86**:547-552. DOI: 10.1136/heart.86.5.547

[12] Khan MF, Athappan G. Left main coronary artery disease. Interventional Cardiology. 2009;**1**:73-91

[13] Leschka S, Alkadhi H, Plass A, Desbiolles L, Grünenfelder J, Marincek B, et al. Accuracy of MSCT coronary angiography with 64-slice technology: First experience. European Heart Journal. *2005*;**26**:1482-1487. DOI: 10.1093/eurheartj/ehi261

[14] Mollet NR, Cademartiri F, van Mieghem CA, Runza G, McFadden EP, Baks T, et al. High-resolution spiral computed tomography coronary angiography in patients referred for diagnostic conventional coronary angiography. Circulation. 2005;**112**:2318-2323. DOI: 10.1161/CIRCULATIONAHA.105.533471

[15] Langer C, Wiemer M, Peterschroder A, Franzke K, Meyer H, Horstkotte D. Images in cardiovascular medicine. Multislice computed tomography and magnetic resonance imaging: Complementary use in noninvasive coronary angiography. Circulation. 2005;**112**: E343-E344. DOI: 10.1161/CIRCULATIONAHA.105.545970

[16] Kallikazaros I, Tsioufis C, Sideris S, Stefanadis C, Toutouzas P. Carotid artery disease as a marker for the presence of severe coronary artery disease in patients evaluated for chest pain. Stroke. 1999;**30**:1002-1007

[17] Hillis LD, Smith PK, Anderson JL, Bittl JA, Bridges CR, Byrne JG, et al. 2011 ACCF/AHA guideline for coronary artery bypass surgery: A report of the American College of Cardiology Foundation/American Heart Association task force on practice guidelines. Circulation. 2011;**124**:e652-e735. DOI: 10.1161/CIR.0b013e31823c074e

[18] The VA Coronary Artery Bypass Surgery Cooperative Study Group. Eighteen-year follow-up in the Veterans Affairs Cooperative Study of coronary artery bypass surgery for stable angina. Circulation 1992;86:121-130.

[19] Varnauskas E. Twelve-year follow-up of survival in the randomized European coronary surgery study. The New England Journal of Medicine. 1988;**319**:332-337

[20] Passamani E, Davis KB, Gillespie MJ, Killip T. A randomized trial of coronary artery bypass surgery. Survival of patients with a low ejection fraction. The New England Journal of Medicine. 1985;**312**:1665-1671

[21] Yusuf S, Zucker D, Peduzzi P, Fisher LD, Takaro T, Kennedy JW, et al. Effect of coronary artery bypass graft surgery on survival: Overview of 10-year results from randomised trials by the coronary artery bypass graft surgery Trialists collaboration. Lancet. 1994;**344**:563-570

[22] Ragosta M. Left main coronary artery disease: Importance, diagnosis, assessment and management. Current Problems in Cardiology. 2015;**40**:93-126. DOI: 10.1016/j.cpcardiol.2014.11.003

[23] Serruys PW, Morice MC, Kappetein AP, Colombo A, Holmes DR, Mack MJ, et al. Percutaneous coronary intervention versus coronary artery bypass grafting for severe coronary artery disease. New England Journal of Medicine. 2209;**360**:961-972. DOI: 10.1056/NEJMoa0804626

[24] Capodanno D, Capranzano P, Di Salvo ME, et al. Usefulness of SYNTAX score to select patients with left main coronary artery disease to be treated with coronary artery bypass graft. JACC Cardiovascular Interventions. 2009;**2**:731-738

[25] Mohr FW, Morice MC, Kappetein AP, Feldman TE, Stahle E, Colombo A, et al. Coronary artery bypass graft surgery versus percutaneous coronary intervention in patients with three-vessel disease and left main coronary disease: 5-year follow-up of the randomized, clinical SYNTAX trial. Lancet. 2013;**381**:629-638. DOI: 10.1016/S0140-6736(13)60141-5

[26] Morice MC, Serruys PW, Kappetein AP, Feldman TE, Stahle E, Colombo A, et al. Five-year outcomes in patients with left main disease treated with either percutaneous coronary intervention or coronary artery bypass grafting in the SYNTAX trial. Circulation. 2014;**129**:2388-2394. DOI: 10.1161/CIRCULATIONAHA.113.006689.

[27] Farooq V, Vergouwe Y, Raber L, Vranckx P, Garcia-Garcia H, Diletti R, et al. Combined anatomical and clinical factors for the long-term risk stratification of patients undergoing

percutaneous coronary intervention: The logistic clinical SYNTAX score. European Heart Journal. 2012;**33**:3098-3104. DOI: 10.1093/eurheartj/ehs295

[28] Farooq V, van Klaveren D, Steyerberg EW, Meliga E, Vergouwe Y, Chieffo A, et al. Anatomical and clinical characteristics to guide decision making between coronary artery bypass surgery and percutaneous coronary intervention for individual patients: Development and validation of SYNTAX score II. Lancet. 2013;**381**(9867):639-650. DOI: 10.1016/S0140-6736(13)60108-7

[29] Shahian DM, O'Brien SM, Filardo G, Ferraris VA, Haan CK, Rich JB, et al. The Society of Thoracic Surgeons 2008 cardiac surgery risk models: Part 1: Coronary artery bypass grafting surgery. The Annals of Thoracic Surgery. 2009;**88**(1 Suppl):S2-22. DOI: 10.1016/j.athoracsur.2009.05.053.

[30] Windecker S, Kolh P, Alfonso F, Collet JP, Cremer J, Falk V, et al. 2014 ESC/EACTS guidelines on myocardial revascularization the task force on myocardial revascularization of the European Society of Cardiology (ESC) and the European Association for Cardio-Thoracic Surgery (EACTS). European Heart Journal. 2014;**35**:2541-2619. DOI: 10.1093/eurheartj/ehu278

[31] O'Keefe JH, Hartzler GO, Rutherford BD, et al. Left main coronary angioplasty. Early and late results of 127 acute and elective procedures. The American Journal of Cardiology. 1989;**64**:144-147

[32] Athappan G, Patvardhan E, Tuzcu ME, Ellis S, Whitlow P, Kapadia SR. Left main coronary artery stenosis. A meta analysis of drug eluting stents versus coronary artery bypass grafting. JACC Cardiovascular Interventions. 2013;**6**:1219-1230. DOI: 10.1016/j.jcin.2013.07.008

[33] Erglis A, Narbute I, Kumsars I, Jegere S, Mintale I, Zakke I, et al. A randomized comparison of paclitaxel-eluting stents versus bare-metal stents for treatment of unprotected left main coronary artery stenosis. Journal of the American College of Cardiology. 2007;**50**:491-497. DOI: 10.1016/j.jacc.2007.03.055

[34] Toyofuku M, Kimura T, Morimoto T, Hayashi Y, Ueda H, Kawai K, et al. Three-year outcomes after sirolimus-eluting stent implantation for unprotected left main coronary artery disease: Insights from the j-Cypher registry. Circulation. 2009;**120**:1866-1874. DOI: 10.1161/CIRCULATIONAHA.109.873349

[35] Valgimigli M, van Mieghem CA, Ong AT, Aoki J, Granillo GA, McFadden EP, et al. Short- and long-term clinical outcome after drug-eluting stent implantation for the percutaneous treatment of left main coronary artery disease: Insights from the Rapamycin-Eluting and Taxus Stent Evaluated At Rotterdam Cardiology Hospital registries (RESEARCH and T-SEARCH). Circulation. 2005;**111**:1383-1389. DOI: 10.1161/01.CIR.0000158486.20865.8B

[36] Mehilli J, Kastrati A, Byrne RA, Bruskina O, Iijima R, Schulz S, et al. Paclitaxel- versus sirolimus-eluting stents for unprotected left main coronary artery disease. Journal of the American College of Cardiology. 2009;**53**:1760-1768. DOI: 10.1016/j.jacc.2009.01.035

[37] Stone GW, Sabik JF, Serruys PW, Simonton CA, Genereux P, Puskas J, et al. Everolimus-eluting stents or bypass surgery for left main coronary artery disease. The New England Journal of Medicine. 2016;**375**:2223-2235. DOI: 10.1056/NEJMoa1610227

[38] Mäkikallio T, Holm NR, Lindsay M, Spence MS, Erglis A, Menown IB, et al. Percutaneous coronary angioplasty versus coronary artery bypass grafting in treatment of unprotected left main stenosis (NOBLE): A prospective, randomised, open-label, non-inferiority trial. Lancet. Dec 3, 2016;**388**(10061):2743-2752. DOI: 10.1016/S0140-6736(16)32052-9

[39] Maziak DE, Rao V, Christakis GT, Buth KJ, Sever J, Fremes SE, et al. Can patients with left main stenosis wait for coronary artery bypass grafting? The Annals of Thoracic Surgery. 1996;**61**:552-557. DOI: 10.1016/0003-4975(95)00835-7

[40] Head SJ, Kaul S, Mack MJ, Serruys PW, Taggart DP, Holmes Jr DR, et al. The rationale for heart team decision-making for patients with stable, complex coronary artery disease. European Heart Journal 2013;**34**: 2510-2518. DOI: 10.1093/eurheartj/eht059

[41] Cohn L, editor. Cardiac Surgery in the Adult, 4th ed. USA: The McGrow Hill Comp.; 2012. 1448 p

[42] Douville EC, Kratz JM, Spinale FG, Crawford Jr FA, Alpert CC, Pearce A. Retrograde versus antegrade cardioplegia: Impact on right ventricular function. The Annals of Thoracic Surgery. 1992;**54**:56-61. DOI: 10.1016/0003-4975(92)91140-5

[43] Onorati F, Renzulli A, De Feo M, Santarpino G, Gregorio R, Biondi A, et al. Does antegrade blood cardioplegia alone provide adequate myocardial protection in patients with left main stem disease? The Journal of Thoracic and Cardiovascular Surgery. 2003; **126**:1345-1351. DOI: 10.1016/S0022

[44] Kouchoukos NT, Blackstone EH, Hanley FL, Kirklin JK, editors. Kirklin/Barratt-Boyes Cardiac Surgery. 4th ed. Philadelphia: Elsevier Saunders; 2013. 2054 p

[45] Sellke FW, DiMaio JM, Caplan LR, Ferguson TB, Gardner TJ, Hiratzka LF, et al. Comparing on-pump and off-pump coronary artery bypass grafting: Numerous studies but few conclusions: A scientific statement from the American Heart Association Council on cardiovascular surgery and Anesthesia in collaboration with the interdisciplinary working group on quality of care and outcomes Research. Circulation. 2005;**111**:2858-2864. DOI: 10.1161/CIRCULATIONAHA.105.165030

[46] Athanasopoulos LV, Athanasiou T. Off-pump coronary artery bypass grafting in left main stem stenosis: Outcomes, concerns and controversies. Journal of Thoracic Disease. 2016;**8**(Suppl 10):s787-s794. DOI: 10.21037/jtd.2016.09.72

[47] Cameron A, Davis KB, Green G, Schaff HV. Coronary bypass surgery with internal-thoracic-artery grafts: Effects on survival over a 15-year period. The New England Journal of Medicine. 1996;**334**:216-219. DOI: 10.1056/NEJM199601253340402

[48] Loop FD, Lytle BW, Cosgrove DM, Stewart RW, Goormastic M, Williams GW, et al. Influence of the internalmammary- artery graft on 10-year survival and other cardiac events. The New England Journal of Medicine. 1986;**314**:1-6. DOI: 10.1056/NEJM-198601023140101

[49] Tatoulis J, Royse AG, Buxton BF, Fuller JA, Skillington PD, Goldblatt JC, et al. The radial artery in coronary surgery: A 5-year experience-clinical and angiographic results. The Annals of Thoracic Surgery. 2002;**73**:143-147

[50] Işık M, Yüksek T, Dereli Y, Görmüş N, Durgut K, Koç O. Evaluation of post-operative flow and diameter changes in brachial and ulnar arteries in coronary artery bypass surgery patients in which the radial artery is used as graft. Türk Kardiyoloji Derneği Arşivi. 2015;**43**:630-636. DOI: 10.5543/tkda.2015.62679

[51] Maniar HS, Sundt TM, Barner HB, Prasad SM, Peterson L, Absi T, et al. Effect of target stenosis and location on radial artery graft patency. The Journal of Thoracic and Cardiovascular Surgery. 2002;**123**:45-52. DOI: 10.1067/mtc.2002.118686

[52] Desai ND, Cohen EA, Naylor CD, Fremes SE, Investigators RAPS. A randomized comparison of radial-artery and saphenous-vein coronary bypass grafts. The New England Journal of Medicine. 2004;**351**:2302-2309. DOI: 10.1056/NEJMoa040982

[53] Bourassa MG, Fisher LD, Campeau L, Gillespie MJ, McConney M, Lesperance J. Long-term fate of bypass grafts: The coronary artery surgery study (CASS) and Montreal heart institute experiences. Circulation. 1985;**72**:V71-V78

Chapter 4

Coronary Artery Bypass Grafting in Patients with Diabetes Mellitus: A Cardiologist's View

Bezdenezhnykh Natalia Alexandrovna,
Sumin Alexei Nikolaevich,
Bezdenezhnykh Andrey Viktorovich and
Barbarash Olga Leonidovna

Additional information is available at the end of the chapter

http://dx.doi.org/10.5772/intechopen.70416

Abstract

The review presents current data on the prevalence of diabetes in the cohort of patients undergoing coronary artery bypass grafting. The relevance of active approach to the identification of diabetes and prediabetes in patients with coronary artery disease (CAD) before coronary revascularization is reviewed. Recent information about the negative impact of diabetes on the prognosis of myocardial revascularization is reported as well as the main mechanisms responsible to the development of adverse outcomes of interventions in these patients. Target perioperative values of glycemia recommended by the leading associations of the study of diabetes have been compared. Beneficial potential of other carbohydrate metabolism markers (glycated hemoglobin, fructosamine, 1,5-anhydroglucitol) in patients with diabetes mellitus (DM) in terms of their impact on cardiovascular prognosis, including coronary intervention. The results of studies comparing different management strategies for these patients are reviewed. The significance of carbohydrate metabolism compensation during myocardial revascularization is reported; thus, a too stringent glycemic control has no benefits neither for percutaneous nor for open coronary intervention. Recent trials suggest the groups of antidiabetic drugs and evidence of their impact on the cardiovascular system. The importance of comprehensive monitoring of major risk factors in diabetic patients with coronary intervention has been proved.

Keywords: diabetes mellitus, prediabetes, early diagnosis of diabetes, ischemic heart disease, coronary artery bypass surgery, percutaneous coronary intervention, myocardial revascularization, target levels of glycemic control, glycated hemoglobin, perioperative antihyperglycemic therapy, perioperative management

1. Introduction

Diabetes mellitus (DM) is one of the most common comorbid conditions in patients with coronary artery disease (CAD), which is important in determining the severity of the disease, treatment strategy, and the prognosis of patients [1].

The increasing prevalence of diabetes has led to a situation where over 380 million people had diabetes mellitus globally in 2013, of whom 99% suffered from type 2 diabetes [2]. According to the population statistics, the number of people present with diabetes is increasing annually. By 2030, this number is expected to rise to more than 550 million people with diabetes and up to 300 million people with prediabetes [2]. This dramatic rise is fuelled mainly by the aging of the population and continuing changes in eating habits and lifestyle with predominant sedentary behavior. In 2014, an estimated 4.9 million deaths were caused by diabetes, of which 60% had the underlying cardiovascular diseases (CVDs) [2].

Therefore, teamwork of cardiologists and endocrinologists is needed to optimally manage diabetes. The efforts of cardiology and diabetes communities have been recently targeted at developing joint guidelines and statements on diabetes management. All current guidelines on management of patients with stable and acute CAD, including guidelines on myocardial revascularization, contain a separate section on diabetes mellitus [3–6], whereas, the guidelines of the International Diabetes Federation, Canadian and American Diabetes Association devote separate sections on cardiovascular diseases (CVD) [7–10]. In 2013, the European Society of Cardiology developed the guidelines on diabetes, prediabetes, and cardiovascular diseases in collaboration with the European Association for the Study of Diabetes [11]. According to the updated guidelines, the search for approaches to optimize the negative impact of diabetes on the results of surgical management remains relevant and includes the study of optimal targets for carbohydrate metabolism, the improvements in the preoperative and perioperative management strategies [7–10]. This review covers the known and insufficiently studied issues of treating patients with diabetes mellitus undergoing myocardial revascularization from the perspective of evidence-based medicine.

2. Prevalence of diabetes in coronary revascularization

The management of CAD patients with concomitant diabetes who need myocardial revascularization is a great challenge. Recent studies demonstrated that a large proportion of CAD patients are present with diabetes [12–15]. The prevalence of diabetes among patients who have undergone percutaneous coronary intervention (PCI) varies greatly from 25 to 30%, according to the DES LATE, ISAR SAFE, RESET, SECURITY trials up to 35–39% in the EXCELLENT, OPTIMIZE, ITALIC, ARCTIC-Interruption trials, and CathPCI Registry [12–14]. The proportion of diabetic patients suffering from CAD undergoing coronary artery bypass grafting accounts for 22–48% of cases [16–20]. In a large Swedish Registry, comprising of 39,235 patients undergoing isolated CABG, 22.8% of patients had diabetes mellitus [18]. The prevalence of diabetes among patients undergoing coronary artery bypass grafting (CABG) is 20–23% according to the results of the Russian studies [20, 21], whereas the US CABG registry suggested the diabetes prevalence to be of 46.9% [19]. A recent Japanese study reported that the proportion of patients with diabetes undergoing direct myocardial revascularization reaches 48% [16].

Differences in diabetes prevalence rates are mainly caused by different diagnostic approaches and racial/ethnic disparities. A large-scale multi-ethnic registry study CREDO-Kyoto comprised 15,580 patients undergoing either CABG or PCI [29]. The lowest rate of diabetes was found in the Caucasian group, whereas the highest ones in the African Americans and the Hispanic group (26.9 vs. 44 vs. 49.5%, respectively). The prevalence rate in the Japanese group was 39% [29].

In addition, several studies confirmed a steady increase in the proportion of diabetic patients undergoing coronary revascularization. In the period from 1999 to 2008, in the Chinese cohort of patients who have undergone CABG, the proportion of diabetic patients increased from 20 to 32% [17], whereas in the American—from 26 to 46% [19]. Moreover, a recent study demonstrated that the rate of diabetes increased by 32% among the patients undergoing CABG [22].

3. Early diagnosis of diabetes in CAD patients undergoing myocardial revascularization

The sharp increase in the prevalence of diabetes among interventional cardiology and cardiac surgery patients is caused by the aging of the population, expanding clinical indications for myocardial revascularization, and recent advances in diagnostic strategies for diabetes and other glycemic disorders [11]. The leading medical associations and communities use the same cut-offs to establish the diagnosis of diabetes mellitus: a fasting plasma glucose concentration ≥ 7.0 and/or 11.1 mmol/l after postglucose load and meal, and/or glycated hemoglobin (HbA1c) >6.5% [7, 8, 10]. However, there are some differences in diagnostic criteria for prediabetes based on fasting glucose and HbA1c. According to the American Diabetes Association (ADA), prediabetes is diagnosed if one or more of the following criteria are met: glycemia of 5.6 mmol/l or HbA1c of 5.7%; whereas the World Health Organization (WHO) implements the following criteria: glucose level of 6.1 mmol/l, or glycated hemoglobin of 6.0% [7, 10].

More rigorous approaches to the diagnosis of carbohydrate metabolism disorders are evident. Type 2 diabetes develops after a long period of euglycemia, but with the existing insulin resistance, which gradually turns into a deficit of beta cells with severe hyperglycemia. The development of CVD in individuals with insulin resistance is a long progressive process. When patients develop hyperglycemia and diagnose type 2 diabetes, 60% of them already have CVD [11, 23, 24].

The guidelines of the American Diabetes Association recommend to assess the glycemic state in adults of any age who are overweight or obese and who have one or more additional risk factors for diabetes (including cardiovascular diseases) and in all people aged >45 years [10]. The European Society of Cardiology and the European Association for the Study of Diabetes recommend if HbA1c and/or fasting plasma glucose (FPG) are inconclusive in individuals with CAD, no diabetes risk score is needed, but an oral glucose tolerance test (OGTT) is indicated [11]. Thus, all patients without previously diagnosed diabetes referred to elective coronary artery bypass grafting should be screened for diabetes or prediabetes.

The rationale for detecting disorders of carbohydrate metabolism has been demonstrated in several studies in patients with CAD, including those undergoing myocardial revascularization. Over 50% of myocardial infarction (MI) patients without known disorders of carbohydrate metabolism had positive OGTT in the in-hospital period [25].

The Spanish trial reported a high prevalence of diabetes up to 45% in patients undergoing PCI, based on continuous OGTT and glycated hemoglobin measurement. Importantly, a third of patients with positive testing were patients who had newly detected diabetes [26]. In their series, 28.8% had known diabetes, 16.2% newly detected diabetes, 25.5% prediabetes, and 29.5% were normoglycemics [26].

Balakrishnan et al. reported 39% of patients with diabetes out of 740 patients admitted to the hospital for PCI. Periprocedural measurement of glycated hemoglobin in patients without known disorders of glucose metabolism allowed to diagnose diabetes and prediabetes in 8.3 and 58.5% of patients, respectively [27].

A prospective Swedish study assessing the prevalence and prognostic impact of the different states of abnormal glucose regulation (AGR) after CABG reported the prevalence of known diabetes of 29.5% [28]. Out of the rest, 11.4% of patients had newly diagnosed diabetes based on oral glucose tolerance test. Thus, the proportion of patients with diabetes increased up to 41%. Another 24% of patients had prediabetes according to the postglucose load. A total of 65% of patients had disorders of carbohydrate metabolism [28].

Why do physicians need to perform active screening for undiagnosed diabetes in patients undergoing cardiac surgeries, and is there any rationale for it? Undiagnosed diabetes may affect the prognosis in this group of patients, similarly to previously diagnosed diabetes [25, 28, 29].

In the EARLY ACS trial of 8795 patients with non-ST-segment elevation ACS, newly diagnosed diabetes was a predictor of 30-day mortality or myocardial infarction [odds ratio (OR) 1.65; confidence interval (CI) 95%; 1.09–2.48] [29]. Previously diagnosed diabetes correlated with a 30-day mortality rate, but not with the MI rate [29].

Similarly, to known disorders of carbohydrate metabolism, newly diagnosed disorders affect the in-hospital and long-term prognosis of patients with myocardial infarction [25]. There was a successive increase in the risk of unfavorable cardiovascular events in the long-term period from normoglycemia through prediabetes to diabetes [28].

4. Benefits of coronary artery bypass grafting over percutaneous coronary intervention and medical therapy in diabetic patients with multivessel coronary artery disease

A sufficient number of studies aimed at choosing an optimal method for myocardial revascularization in patients with diabetes have been performed [30–37]. A large BARI-2D trial focused at assessing myocardial revascularization in patients with diabetes with stable coronary artery disease [30, 31]. Patients selected for the CABG stratum had more extensive coronary artery disease. Nevertheless, the rate of major cardiovascular events was significantly lower in the revascularization group, compared with the medical therapy group [30, 31].

The revascularization group patients demonstrated fewer cases of angina progression (8 vs. 13%, respectively, $p < 0.001$), recurrent angina (37 vs. 51%, respectively, $p < 0.001$), and subsequent coronary revascularization, compared to the intensive medical management group (18 vs. 33%, respectively, $p < 0.001$) [31]. The revascularization group patients exhibited a trend toward being angina-free at 3-year follow-up than the intensive medical management group (66 vs. 58%, respectively, $p < 0.003$). The superiority of revascularization strategy over medical therapy is believed to be caused by preferring CABG over PCI in patients with more severe coronary artery disease [31].

The FREEDOM (future revascularization evaluation in patients with diabetes mellitus) study is a single, well-powered, randomized trial, comparing CABG and PCI with first-generation drug-eluting stent (DES) (94%) in diabetic patients undergoing elective revascularization for multivessel coronary disease without left main coronary artery stenosis [33]. The rate of the primary outcome was lower in the CABG group than in the PCI group, with divergence of the curves starting at 2 years. This difference was due to a relative reduction in death from any cause ($p = 0.049$) and a significantly lower incidence of MI in the CABG group ($p < 0.001$) [33].

A review of 13 RCTs and 5 meta-analyses agreed that CABG surgery should be recommended in patients with diabetes and multivessel CAD, regardless of the severity of coronary anatomy: CABG improved the long-term prognosis. Thus, the 5-year risk of major cardiovascular events was 18.7% in the CABG group vs. 26.6% in the PCI group, $p = 0.005$) [34].

A recent meta-analysis of six RCTs showed similar results, confirming the benefits of direct revascularization over PCI in patients with diabetes. CABG was associated with a significantly lower mortality, compared with PCI (RR: 0.59, 95% CI 0.42–0.85; $p = 0.004$). The rates of major cardiovascular and cerebrovascular events, as well as repeat revascularization, were significantly lower in the CABG group (OR 0.51, 95% CI 0.27–0.99, $p = 0.03$ vs. OR 0.34, 95% CI 0.24–0.49; $p < 0.00001$, respectively) [35].

Since available data suggesting beneficial effects of myocardial revascularization in patients with diabetes were obtained in the period of advancements in pharmacotherapy and technology of both PCI and surgical revascularization, it is difficult to compare them directly. Nevertheless, many studies have shown that CABG appears to be a better option compared to PCI with DES in diabetic patients, particularly, if the patient has multivessel CAD [33–37]. The superiority of coronary artery bypass grafting over percutaneous coronary intervention in diabetic patients with multivessel coronary disease is currently stated in the international guidelines with the class of recommendation IA [5].

5. Diabetes mellitus and outcomes of myocardial revascularization

Although diabetic patients constitute an increasing number of individuals undergoing PCI and surgical revascularization, they have worse outcomes, than non-diabetic patients [14,

37–39]. The meta-analysis of several randomized clinical trials of coronary angioplasty using bare-metal stents has proved diabetes to be the strongest predictor of restenosis, with a high risk of repeat revascularization of the target lesion [37]. In multivariable analyses of 6081 patients undergoing PCI with the implantation of DES, diabetic vs. non-diabetic patients had higher risks of major adverse cardiac events (odds ratio (OR), 1.25; 95% confidence interval (CI), 1.03–1.53; $p = 0.026$), but similar risks of cardiac death (OR, 1.41; 95% CI, 0.96–2.07; $p = 0.08$) and myocardial infarction (OR, 0.89; 95% CI, 0.64–1.22; $p = 0.45$) [38].

The two major causes of stent failure are stent thrombosis and in-stent restenosis. The incidence of both has reduced considerably in recent years [14]. Current clinical registries and randomized trials with broad inclusion criteria show rates of stent thrombosis at or <1% after 1 year; rates of clinical in-stent restenosis are 5%, respectively [12–14]. Angiographic surveillance studies in large cohorts show rates of angiographic in-stent restenosis of ~10% with new-generation DES [14]. However, the contribution of diabetes to the development of restenosis remains significant. One of the largest analysis, comprising of 10,004 patients with completed angiographic follow-up after PCI found that diabetes mellitus was an independent predictor of restenosis (OR 1.32, 95% CI 1.19–1.46), as well as previous CABG, complex lesion morphology, smaller vessel reference diameter before the procedure, and greater stented length of the vessel [14]. Angiographic follow-up of 123 patients after PCI demonstrated that DM was associated with a 3-fold increased risk of plaque neovascularization. Importantly, more than half of the patients (56.5%) failed to reach the target range of glycated hemoglobin [40].

There is a strong association between diabetes and high rates of complications after CABG. Despite the fact that in-hospital mortality rates among diabetic patients significantly decreased from 3% in the period 1998–2002 to 1.3% in the period 2003–2005 [35], postoperative complication rates remain high. Thus, a retrospective analysis, comprising 667 CAD patients, who have undergone CABG, showed that diabetes did not affect in-hospital mortality, but was an independent predictor of sternal wound infection [41]. Similar findings were obtained in another retrospective study, suggesting the absence of any correlations between diabetes and the risk of cardiovascular complications and mortality. However, the obtained findings revealed a significant association between diabetes and renal complication after CABG [42]. Diabetic patients have poor immediate outcomes after CABG and unfavorable long-term prognosis, compared to non-diabetic patients. Moreover, patients with diabetes had higher rates of the hospitalization and major cardiovascular events [18, 28, 43]. A recent Russian study with the 5-year follow-up period reported that 14.2% of patients with diabetes had one of the major cardiovascular events (myocardial infarction, stroke, or cardiovascular death) vs. 6.3% patients without diabetes ($p = 0.028$) [39]. Despite new insights into pathophysiology of diabetes and recent improvements in the perioperative management, DM remains a challenging issue for coronary procedures and interventions.

6. Diabetes-specific risk factors for adverse prognosis in coronary procedures and interventions

Adverse prognosis in this group of patients is partially explained by initial characteristics of diabetic patients referred to elective revascularization. These patients commonly have higher perioperative risk due to advanced age, obesity, female gender, previous cardiovascular events and revascularization procedures, multivessel coronary disease, severe heart failure, chronic kidney disease, and chronic obstructive pulmonary disease. These conditions are known to independently affect the prognosis of patients with CAD [5, 23]. In addition, diabetic patients are more likely to have multivessel coronary disease, diffuse coronary lesions, poor distal vascular bed, and calcification [5].

However, there are diabetes-specific factors, namely hyperglycemia, insulin resistance, and hyperinsulinemia, which cause a cascade of pathogenetic reactions [44]. Thus, diabetic patients have more intense intravascular inflammation than non-diabetic ones. Excess pro-inflammatory cytokines and other biologically active substances lead to the destabilization of an atherosclerotic plaque, the progression of coronary atherosclerosis to unaffected segments of the vascular wall [44, 45]. Moreover, the analysis reported a diminished numerical density of mast cells and a significantly higher volume density of the mononuclear cells [46]. Hyperglycemia can lead to the development of endothelial dysfunction, associated with reduced nitric oxide, a key signaling regulator of vascular tone, and increased oxidative stress. In addition, acute hyperglycemia worsens insulin activity in endothelial cells even at physiologically adequate levels [23].

A prospective study, comprising of 1035 patients with myocardial infarction, who have undergone primary PCI in one of the Chinese hospitals, found a relationship between acute hyperglycemia at the time of admission and poor short- and long-term prognosis [47]. Pre- and postoperative hyperglycemia is the main risk factor for developing infectious complications after CABG in both diabetic and non-diabetic patients [41]. Hyperglycemia is associated with impaired leukocyte function, including diminished chemotaxis, decreased phagocytosis, impaired bacterial killing, and abnormal adhesive properties [44]. Diabetic patients showed higher endothelial activation and lower antiinflammatory response to CPB compared to non-diabetics [46]. Chronic hyperglycemia can lead to the central nervous system injury, resulting in diabetic encephalopathy with the onset of mild and moderate cognitive disorders [48]. Bruce et al. found that 64% of diabetic patients with coronary artery disease had cognitive or emotional disorders [49].

In addition, diabetes mellitus is a predictor of increased aggregation potential. SP-selectin, intercellular adhesion molecules, and platelet aggregation were significantly higher in diabetic patients, than in non-diabetics [44]. Despite receiving the same dose of aspirin and clopidogrel, patients with diabetes had higher values of platelet reactivity according to the findings of the recent study evaluating the effects of double antiplatelet therapy in diabetic patients with stable coronary artery disease [46]. Periprocedural control of glycemia in patients undergoing coronary interventions is pivotal for both endocrinologists and cardiologists. The current guidelines of the Canadian Diabetes Association (CDA) state that patients with diabetes do not receive the necessary glycemic control when they are admitted to non-profile hospitals [8].

7. Perioperative target glycemic range for myocardial revascularization and the risk of hypoglycemia

The current national guidelines, based on evidence-based medicine, have regulated the perioperative target range of glycemia [7–10]. The target range of glycemia for the majority of ICU patients, defined by the International Diabetes Federation, the American and Canadian Diabetes Associations, are the following: 140–180 mg/dL without hypoglycemia and 80–180 mg/dL for the perioperative period [8, 10].

All guidelines strictly recommend to avoid hypoglycemia. The risk of developing hypoglycemia inevitably increases with the attempts to achieve compensation for carbohydrate metabolism. Therefore, many studies, suggesting beneficial effects of perioperative glucose control, did not confirm their hypothesis [50–53]. A tighter control did not show its superiority neither for the immediate outcomes after CABG [50, 51], nor for the long-term outcomes [52]. Intensive insulin therapy with the achievement of perioperative target glucose levels of 100–140 (5.5–7.7 mmol/l) after CABG does not significantly reduce the number of postoperative complications, compared with the target glucose level of 140–170 (7.8–9.2 mmol/l) [51, 53].

A scientific statement from the American Diabetes Association and the American Heart Association Society suggests that severe hypoglycemia is the most likely cause of increased cardiovascular mortality in diabetic patients with intensive control of glycemia [54]. Unfortunately, hypoglycemia is more likely to happen when blood glucose decrease up to physiological values.

Hypoglycemia commonly develops with intensive insulin therapy, and is a well-known risk factor for MI, stroke, and death from any causes [53]. The relative risk for developing MI, associated with severe hypoglycemia 1 year before the index event, was 12%, 5.5 months before MI—20%, and 2 weeks before—65% [55].

Hypoglycemia triggers a powerful stimulation of the autonomic nervous system and the excess release of catecholamines, which promote vasospasm, tachycardia, arterial hypertension, and increased blood viscosity and coagulation [56]. These processes may cause changes in the regional blood flow and provoke myocardial or cerebral ischemia, resulting in myocardial infarction, heart failure, or stroke. Unfortunately, similar to fatal events, it is very difficult to demonstrate any relationship between severe hypoglycemia and serious vascular events, since clinical evidence of the impact of hypoglycemia are mainly random [55]. Death caused by hypoglycemia can be mistaken for death from acute coronary syndrome, because no one measures glycemia before. There are no anatomical and morphological postmortem signs of hypoglycemia [55, 56].

Withholding glucose in the target range without hypoglycemia and its impact on the prognosis are highly relevant issues for further research, as well as the use of integrated glucose metabolism indicators, such as glycated hemoglobin, which may improve the comprehensive risk assessment of surgical intervention.

8. Glycated hemoglobin and outcomes of coronary procedures and interventions

Glycated hemoglobin (HbA1c) is used for monitoring blood glucose levels in diabetic patients; it should be measured in all diabetic patients once in 3 months, and before any surgical interventions, including coronary revascularization. A systematic review of 11 studies addressing the relationship between glycated hemoglobin levels and the results of CABG in diabetic and non-diabetic patients was performed [57]. Four studies found significant increase in early and late mortality at higher HbA1c levels, regardless of a preoperative diagnosis of diabetes. In particular, the mortality risk for CABG is quadrupled at HbA1c levels >8.6% [57]. However, four studies of early mortality outcomes in diabetic patients only showed no significant differences between patients with normal and those with deranged HbA1c levels ($p = 0.99$). Three studies identified a significant increase in infectious complications in patients with poorly controlled HbA1c: superficial sternal wound infection ($p = 0.014$ and 0.007, respectively) and minor infections ($p = 0.006$) [57].

Unexpected data were obtained in one of the Japanese surgical clinics. Elevated HbA1c was associated with a lower incidence of arrhythmias after CABG. The incidence of postoperative atrial fibrillation was 28.3% in the lower tertile, 17.4% in the middle tertile, and 12.5% in the upper tertile [58]. Thus, the mean and high levels of glycated hemoglobin were associated with a lower incidence of atrial arrhythmias. One possible explanation is that patients with elevated HbA1c require more insulin, which has been reported to reduce the risk of postoperative atrial fibrillation [58]. Similar results were obtained in the recent American study. The incidence of atrial fibrillation after CABG was 20.9% in patients with HbA1c < 7.0% and 15.1% in patients with HbA1c ≥ 7.0% ($p = 0.007$), adjusted OR 0.73; 95% CI 0.55–0.96 [57]. However, elevated HbA1c was associated with higher rates of postoperative stroke, renal failure, and deep wound infection [57].

Some studies have called into question the predictive potential of HbA1c for short-term outcomes in well-controlled diabetics. However, poor control and elevated HbA1c may result in high rate of adverse events in the short- and long-term postoperative periods [57, 59].

Maintaining a level of glycemia close to the physiological level is an achievable goal of hypoglycemic therapy in type 2 diabetes. Its significance is evident and is associated with the risk of developing specific chronic complications induced by hyperglycemia. However, appropriate glycemic control with glucose levels closer to normal is associated with a high risk of hypoglycemia, which is known to affect the prognosis in diabetic patients with CVD [56]. Therefore, the search and development of optimal and safe tools to manage high glucose levels are pivotal for modern medical research.

9. The degree of compensation of carbohydrate metabolism and long-term prognosis in patients with diabetes and coronary artery disease

The UKPDS study was the first one to demonstrate the significance of the compensation of carbohydrate metabolism for the progression of complications [60]. The obtained results stimulated other researches in this area addressed to the assessment of the control intensity in patients with CVD, but the obtained data did not show the superiority of the tight strategy [61–63].

Three major studies (ACCORD, ADVANCE, and VADT) evaluated the impact of attaining euglycemia (ACCORD) or near-euglycemia (ADVANCE, VADT) in older patients with diabetes and high cardiovascular risk [61–63]. None of these studies, either individually or on pooled analysis, demonstrated any reduction in cardiovascular or all-cause mortality with tight glucose control [60]. A higher mortality was observed in the intensive glucose control arm of ACCORD, resulting in the premature termination of the glucose-lowering component of this study. Also, the occurrence of hypoglycemic episodes (total and major) was significantly higher in the intensive glucose control arms of all three studies [60].

The Diabetes Control and Complications Trial (DCCT) and the Epidemiology of Diabetes Interventions and Complications (EDIC) study, DCCT's long-term follow-up study, were aimed at assessing the rate of micro- and macrovascular complications in diabetic patients and their relationships with hypoglycemic therapy. In the DCCT study, the incidence of cardiovascular events was not significantly associated with intensive insulin therapy. 93% of the original cohort of the DCCT study agreed to join the EDIC study with an 11-year follow-up period. The obtained results proved that intensive treatment was associated with reduced risk of any cardiovascular events by 42% during the 17-year follow-up ($p < 0.01$). Thus, DCCT (EDIC), and UKPDS showed that glycemic control in diabetic patients is important for the prevention of microvascular complications, but long-term follow-up is needed to demonstrate these effects [11].

In 2015, the American Diabetes Association and The European Association for the Study of Diabetes updated the positioned statement on the management of hyperglycemia of 2012, suggesting the need for strengthening the patient-centered approach to the management of diabetic patients [64]. They highlighted the necessity to individualize the range for glycemic control. They recommend to use the HbA1c range of 7.5–8% for elderly patients with diabetes and patients with a positive history of cardiovascular events, depending on their life expectancy, age, and social status [64]. A more tight target range (HbA1c 6.5–7.0%) may be used in patients with slow-onset diabetes, long life expectancy, and those without significant cardiovascular disease (CVD), if it can be achieved without hypoglycemia [64].

What tools may be used to control glycemia in patients undergoing myocardial revascul arization?

10. Hypoglycemic therapy in patients undergoing myocardial revascularization—the lack of evidence

A number of new classes of drugs for the treatment of diabetes and their effects on cardiovascular system have been studied well. However, there are limited data regarding in-hospital hypoglycemic therapy in patients undergoing myocardial revascularization. The concerns of medical community on this issue may be found directly in the headlines of recently published manuscripts. Hoogwerf addressed this issue in his article entitled "Perioperative management of diabetes mellitus: how should we act on the limited evidence?" [65]. Despite the fact that this article was published 10 years ago, and during this period new knowledge and evidence have been obtained, the question regarding optimal medical management of glycemia in patients undergoing coronary revascularization remains crucial. Recent guidelines on the management of diabetes [7–10] state the lack of evidence for using non-insulin hypoglycemic drugs in the perioperative period in diabetic patients.

Insulin remains the only approved perioperative method of hypoglycemic therapy. The current guidelines recommend use of basal insulin or basal-bolus regimen, and strongly discourage use of sliding-scale while a sliding schedule is strongly discouraged [8, 10].

Continuous intravenous insulin infusion is recognized as the preferred method for achieving and maintaining the glycemic control in critically ill patients [8–10]. The protocols for insulin infusion have been already developed and approved by diabetic communities [8–10]. They allow to adjust the rate of insulin infusion according to the glycemic levels. Insulin therapy should be initiated to treat persistent hyperglycemia, starting at a threshold of 180 mg/dL (10 mmol/L). Episodes of hypoglycemia should be noted in medical records and strictly monitored, since glucose level of 70 mg/dL require the changing of treatment regimen [8–10].

The multicenter DIGAMI, DIGAMI 2, HI-5 trials studied the intensity of the glucose control in ACS patients, including those undergoing PCI. Initially, DIGAMI reported low mortality in MI patients enrolled in the insulin therapy group [66]. However, the follow-up DIGAMI 2 trial with a double sample size and a more careful design did not show any advantages in the group of patients receiving intensive insulin therapy. Moreover, there were no significant differences in the rate of the composite endpoint (cardiovascular death/nonfatal myocardial infarction/stroke) between the intensive control group and the standard therapy group. The HI-5 study received similar results [66]. Since neither the DIGAMI 2, nor the HI-5 achieved differences in the control of glucose between the intensive management group and the control group, the effectiveness of insulin therapy for lowering glucose levels in ACS patients remains controversial. Combined data from these three studies confirmed that glucose-insulin-potassium infusion did not reduce mortality without the glucose control in diabetic patients with ACS (OR 1.07, 95% CI 0.85–1.36, $p = 0.547$) [66]. None of the protocols noted the improvements of the outcomes in patients with ST-segment elevation ACS after PCI, who received insulin or the intravenous glucose-insulin-potassium infusions [66].

The Japanese study, comprising 2148 patients who underwent PCI in the period from 2003 to 2012, showed an association between insulin use and increased rates of myocardial infarction and stent thrombosis [67]. The subgroup analysis of the FREEDOM trial, aimed at assessing outcomes of diabetic patients undergoing either CABG or PCI, reported that patients receiving insulin had a higher rate of major cardiovascular events [68]. Nevertheless, the use of insulin may be regarded as a marker of the severity and duration of diabetes, and does not reflect the true effects of therapy on the outcomes.

Currently, the discontinuation of long-acting drugs before surgical procedures is preferable, but there is no consensus on PCI, since the management of patients is commonly regulated by the local protocol [69]. There are available data suggesting safe and beneficial effects of long-acting oral hypoglycemic agents in PCI patients, resulting in better glycemic control and lower platelet activity [66].

The American and Canadian Diabetes Associations recommend to withhold metformin 24–48 h prior to CAG or PCI, and restart it 48 h after the procedure in the absence of significantly decreased GFR or later after the normalization of renal function [8, 10]. Although, recent studies showed the safety of continuing metformin therapy during the procedure, their statistical capacity is insufficient to change the current guidelines [10, 70, 71].

The recent study of patients with metabolic syndrome who received metformin for 7 days before PCI vs. the placebo group reported a lower rate of perioperative myocardial damage, estimated by elevated creatine phosphokinase-MB ($p = 0.008$) and troponin I ($p = 0.005$). According to the assessment of the 1-year prognosis, the incidence of major cardiovascular events (heart attack/stroke/cardiovascular death) was significantly lower in the metformin group (7.9 and 28.9%, respectively, $p = 0.001$) [72].

A randomized trial of 100 patients who received either 1000 mg of metformin or placebo after CABG in addition to standard insulin therapy, the metformin therapy was initiated 3 h after extubation and lasted for 3 days [70]. Based on the results, the mean dose of insulin, as well as the mean number of episodes of both hyper- and hypoglycemia, were significantly lower in the metformin group ($p < 0.05$). At the same time, the risk of acidosis in the metformin group did not increase [70].

There were some attempts to use metformin in non-diabetic patients undergoing coronary artery bypass grafting. The researchers concluded that the short-term use of metformin prior to CABG was relatively safe, but ineffective strategy for reducing periprocedural myocardial damage in non-diabetic patients [71].

The updated ADA 2017 guidelines noted that the SGLT2 inhibitors, despite their proven cardiovascular effects, cannot yet be recommended for the hospital use, and, therefore, should be avoided before surgical interventions [10].

11. Comprehensive risk factor control in diabetic patients in coronary procedures and interventions

In addition to the compensation of carbohydrate metabolism, multiple monitoring of risk factors in diabetic patients undergoing revascularization should be implemented and include achieving target levels of blood pressure (BP) and lipids, smoking cessation. The BARI-2D trial, focused at assessing coronary revascularization in diabetic patients, reported that both, the tight control over the main risk factors and intensive treatment management in diabetic patients according to the current guidelines, were associated with improved cardiovascular outcomes [23]. Based on the results of the study with a 20-year follow-up after CABG, long-term survival, and freedom from major cardiovascular events in diabetic patients followed CABG was lower. However, the monitoring of carbohydrate metabolism and other risk factors (target levels of lipids and arterial blood pressure, smoking cessation) appears to be significant for the prognosis in this group of patients [43]. Despite the improvements in achieving the goals of treatment for diabetes, it requires further control and monitoring, as only 14.3% of adult Americans with type 2 diabetes have target levels of HbA1c, blood pressure, and low-density lipoprotein cholesterol (LDL-C) [73].

To date, the evidence-based results of randomized clinical trials suggest that statin therapy reduces the incidence of cardiovascular events in diabetic patients [74, 75]. The protective cardiovascular effects of statins significantly outweigh the associated risk of developing diabetes mellitus [75]. The recent joint guidelines of the American Society of Cardiology and the Heart Association recognize diabetic patients aged 40–75 years as one of the four main groups of patients who would most likely benefit from statin therapy [23]. The guidelines of the American and European Society of Cardiologists recommend to initiate statin therapy in all patients who had myocardial infarction, regardless of the cholesterol level [76]. However, there are several studies reporting that low levels of low-density lipoprotein cholesterol (LDL cholesterol), regardless of hypolipidemic therapy, are associated with increased in-hospital mortality in ACS patients, including those undergoing PCI. The results of a study, comprising of 9032 patients with myocardial infarction who underwent primary PCI in 68 centers in Tokyo, convincingly showed that statin therapy significantly reduced in-hospital mortality, even in patients with low LDL cholesterol and those with diabetes [77].

A large retrospective analysis, including 16,192 patients undergoing CABG, demonstrated that the use of statins, regardless of diabetes and other risk factors, was associated with a significant reduction of in-hospital mortality in five logistic regression models [78]. Importantly, angiotensin-converting enzyme (ACE) inhibitors, beta-blockers, and calcium antagonists did not show any significant correlations with the outcomes followed CABG [78]. However, there are available data on beneficial effects of statins on reducing the incidence of atrial fibrillation and cognitive impairment after CABG, including patients with diabetes mellitus [48, 78].

Undoubtedly, patients with diabetes, undergoing revascularization, need to achieve the target levels of systolic blood pressure < 140 mm Hg and diastolic blood pressure < 90 mm Hg. These target levels are required to reduce cardiovascular risk according to the recent statement of the American Heart Association and American Diabetics Association. Moreover, the AHA/ADA guidelines recommend to use ACE inhibitors and angiotensin II receptor antagonists for treating arterial hypertension in diabetic patients [54].

Thus, we may conclude that the negative impact of diabetes on the prognosis after myocardial revascularization and the need to achieve the target ranges of carbohydrate metabolism, as well as the comprehensive cardiovascular control are evident in treating diabetic patients. However, the benefits of the intensive glycemic management remain controversial. Other treatment strategies, such as continuing prescribed hypoglycemic drugs, including long-acting ones, should be considered only in patients undergoing PCI, but not in those who are referred to elective open-heart surgeries. Currently, the issues that require further research have been highlighted in our review and, in a few years, new clinical trials will provide new insights for medical community dealing with diabetes and coronary artery diseases.

Author details

Bezdenezhnykh Natalia Alexandrovna[1]*, Sumin Alexei Nikolaevich[1], Bezdenezhnykh Andrey Viktorovich[1] and Barbarash Olga Leonidovna[1,2]

*Address all correspondence to: n_bez@mail.ru

1 Federal State Budgetary Institution, Research Institute for Complex Issues of Cardiovascular Diseases, Kemerovo, Russian Federation

2 Federal State Budgetary Institution of Higher Professional Education, Kemerovo State Medical Institution, Kemerovo, Russian Federation

References

[1] Inohara T, Kohsaka S, Goto M, et al. Hypothesis of long-term outcome after coronary revascularization in Japanese patients compared to multiethnic groups in the US. PLoS One. 2015;**10**(5):e0128252. DOI: 10.1371/journal.pone.0128252

[2] Guariguata L, Whiting DR, Hambleton I, et al. Global estimates of diabetes prevalence for 2013 and projections for 2035. Diabetes Research and Clinical Practice. 2014;**103**:137-149

[3] Task Force Members, Montalescot G, Sechtem U, Achenbach S, et al. 2013 ESC guidelines on the management of stable coronary artery disease. European Heart Journal. 2013;**34**:2949-3003. DOI: 10.1093/eurheartj/eht296

[4] Task Force on the management of ST-segment elevation acute myocardial infarction of the European Society of Cardiology (ESC), Steg PG, James SK, Atar D, et al. ESC Guidelines for the management of acute myocardial infarction in patients presenting with ST-segment elevation. European Heart Journal. 2012;**33**:2569-2619. DOI: 10.1093/eurheartj/ehs215

[5] Authors/Task Force members, Windecker S, Kolh P, Alfonso F, et al. Guidelines on myocardial revascularization: The task force on myocardial revascularization of the European Society of Cardiology (ESC) and the European Association for Cardio-Thoracic Surgery (EACTS) developed with the special contribution of the European Association of Percutaneous Cardiovascular Interventions (EAPCI). European Heart Journal. 2014;**35**:2541-2619

[6] Patel MR, Calhoon JH, Dehmer GJ, Grantham JA, Maddox TM, Maron DJ, Smith PK. ACC/AATS/AHA/ASE/ASNC/SCAI/SCCT/STS 2017 appropriate use criteria for coronary revascularization in patients with stable ischemic heart disease. Coronary Revascularization Writing Group. Journal of the American College of Cardiology. 2017;**69**:2212-2241. DOI: 10.1016/j.jacc.2017.02.001

[7] International Diabetes Federation. Global Guideline for Type 2 Diabetes [Internet]. 2012. Available from: http://www.idf.org

[8] Canadian Diabetes Association. 2013 clinical practice guidelines for the prevention and management of diabetes in Canada. Canadian Journal of Diabetes. 2013;**37**(1):1-216

[9] Dedov II, Shestakova MV. Standards of specialized diabetes care. 7th edition (Russian). Diabetes mellitus. 2017;**20**(1S):1-112. DOI: 10.14341/DM20171S8

[10] Standards of medical care in diabetes 2017: Summary of revisions. Diabetes Care. 2017;**40**(Suppl. 1):S1-S2. DOI: 10.2337/dc17-S001

[11] Authors/Task Force Members, Rydén L, Grant PJ, Anker SD, et al. ESC Guidelines on diabetes, pre-diabetes, and cardiovascular diseases developed in collaboration with the EASD: The task force on diabetes, pre-diabetes, and cardiovascular diseases of the European Society of Cardiology (ESC) and developed in collaboration with the European Association for the Study of Diabetes (EASD). European Heart Journal. 2013;**34**(39):3035-3087

[12] Schulz-Schüpke S, Byrne RA, ten Berg JM, et al. ISAR-SAFE: A randomized, double-blind, placebo-controlled trial of 6 versus 12 months of clopidogrel therapy after drug-eluting stenting. European Heart Journal. 2015;**36**:1252-1263

[13] Colombo A, Chieffo A, Frasheri A, Garbo R, et al. Second-generation drug-eluting stent implantation followed by 6- versus 12-month dual antiplatelet therapy: The SECURITY randomized clinical trial. Journal of the American College of Cardiology. 2014;**64**:2086-2097

[14] Byrne RA, Joner M, Kastrati A. Stent thrombosis and restenosis: What have we learned and where are we going? The Andreas Grüntzig Lecture ESC 2014. European Heart Journal. 2015;**36**:3320-3331. DOI: 10.1093/eurheartj/ehv511

[15] Tarasov RS, Kochergin AM, Ganiukov VI, et al. The results of endovascular revascularization in elderly patients with myocardial infarction and ST-segment elevation in multivessel lesion depending on the severity of coronary atherosclerosis (Russian). Terapevticheskij Arkhiv. 2016;**88**(1):23-29

[16] Shimizu T, Miura S, Takeuchi K, et al. Effects of gender and aging in patients who undergo coronary artery bypass grafting: From the FU-Registry. Cardiology Journal. 2012;**19**(6):618-624. DOI: 10.5603/CJ.2012.0114

[17] Zhang H, Yuan X, Osnabrugge RL, et al. Influence of diabetes mellitus on long-term clinical and economic outcomes after coronary artery bypass grafting. The Annals of Thoracic Surgery. 2014;**97**(6):2073-2079

[18] Holzmann MJ, Rathsman B, Eliasson B, et al. Long-term prognosis in patients with type 1 and 2 diabetes mellitus after coronary artery bypass grafting. Journal of the American College of Cardiology. 2015;**65**(16):1644-1652. DOI: 10.1016/j.jacc.2015.02.052

[19] D'Agostino RS, Jacobs JP, Badhwar V, et al. The Society of Thoracic Surgeons Adult Cardiac Surgery Database: 2016 update on outcomes and quality. The Annals of Thoracic Surgery. 2016;**101**(1):24-32. DOI: 10.1016/j.athoracsur.2015.11.032

[20] Akchurin RS, Vlasova EE, Mershin KV. Diabetus mellitus and surgical treatment of coronary heart disease (Russian). Annals of the Russian Academy of Medical Sciences. 2012;**1**:14-19

[21] Borodashkina SY, Podkamenny VA, Protasov KV. Cardiovascular complications and carbohydrate metabolism in coronary shunting "off-pump" according to the regimen of glucose lowering treatment in ischemic heart disease and diabetes (Russian). Russian Journal of Cardiology. 2016;**2**:19-24. DOI: 10.15829/1560-4071-2016-2-19-24

[22] Kindo M, Hoang Minh T, Perrier S, Bentz J, Mommerot A, Billaud P, Mazzucotelli JP. Trends in isolated coronary artery bypass grafting over the last decade. Interactive Cardiovascular and Thoracic Surgery. 2017;**24**(1):71-76. DOI: 10.1093/icvts/ivw319 Epub 2016 Sept. 22

[23] Wang CL, Hess CN, Hiatt WR, et al. Clinical update: Cardiovascular disease in diabetes mellitus: Atherosclerotic cardiovascular disease and heart failure in type 2 diabetes mellitus—Mechanisms, management, and clinical considerations. Circulation. 2016;**133**:2459-2502

[24] Romeo GR, Lee J, Shoelson SE, et al. Metabolic syndrome, insulin resistance and roles of inflammation: Mechanisms and therapeutic targets. Arteriosclerosis, Thrombosis, and Vascular Biology. 2012;**32**:1771-1776

[25] Belenkova YA, Karetnikova VN, Dyachenko AO, et al. Inflammation's role in the development of poor prognosis in patients with myocardial infarction-segment elevation ST, undergoing percutaneous coronary intervention, against the background of impaired glucose tolerance and diabetes mellitus (Russian). Russian Cardiology Journal. 2014;**8**(112):84-91

[26] de la Hera JM, Delgado E, Hernández E, et al. Prevalence and outcome of newly detected diabetes in patients who undergo percutaneous coronary intervention. European Heart Journal 2009;**30**(21):2614-2621. DOI: 10.1093/eurheartj/ehp278

[27] Balakrishnan R, Berger JS, Tully L, et al. Prevalence of unrecognized diabetes, prediabetes and metabolic syndrome in patients undergoing elective percutaneous coronary intervention. Diabetes/Metabolism Research and Reviews. 2015;**31**(6):603-609. DOI: 10.1002/dmrr.264

[28] Petursson P, Herlitz J, Lindqvist J, et al. Prevalence and severity of abnormal glucose regulation and its relation to long-term prognosis after coronary artery bypass grafting. Coronary Artery Disease. 2013;**24**(7):577-582

[29] Giraldez RR, Clare RM, Lopes RD, et al. Prevalence and clinical outcomes of undiagnosed diabetes mellitus and prediabetes among patients with high-risk non-ST-segment elevation acute coronary syndrome. American Heart Journal. 2013;**165**(6):918.e2-925.e2. DOI: 10.1016/j.ahj.2013.01.005

[30] Frye RL, August P, Brooks MM, et al. A randomized trial of therapies for type 2 diabetes and coronary artery disease. The New England Journal of Medicine. 2009;**360**(24):2503-2515

[31] Shaw LJ, Cerqueira MD, Brooks MM, et al. Impact of left ventricular function and the extent of ischemia and scar by stress myocardial perfusion imaging on prognosis and therapeutic risk reduction in diabetic patients with coronary artery disease: Results from the bypass angioplasty revascularization investigation 2 diabetes (BARI 2D) trial. Journal of Nuclear Cardiology. 2012;**19**(4):658-669

[32] Brooks MM, Chaitman BR, Nesto RW, et al. Clinical, angiographic risk stratification differential impact on treatment outcomes in the bypass angioplasty revascularization investigation 2 diabetes (BARI 2D) trial. Circulation. 2012;**126**(17):2115-2124

[33] Farkouh ME, Domanski M, Sleeper LA, et al. Strategies for multivessel revascularization in patients with diabetes. The New England Journal of Medicine. 2012;**367**:2375-2384

[34] Deb S, Wijeysundera HC, Ko DT, et al. Coronary artery bypass graft surgery vs. percutaneous interventions in coronary revascularization: A systematic review. Journal of the American Medical Association. 2013;**310**(19):2086-2095. DOI: 10.1001/jama.2013.281718

[35] Bundhun PK, Wu ZJ, Chen M-H. Coronary artery bypass surgery compared with percutaneous coronary interventions in patients with insulin-treated type 2 diabetes mellitus: A systematic review and meta-analysis of 6 randomized controlled trials. Cardiovascular Diabetology. 2016;**15**:2. DOI: 10.1186/s12933-015-0323-z

[36] Bangalore S. Outcomes with coronary artery bypass graft surgery versus percutaneous coronary intervention for patients with diabetes mellitus: Can newer generation drug-eluting stents bridge the gap? Circulation. Cardiovascular Interventions. 2014;**7**(4):518-525

[37] Luthra S, Leiva-Juárez MM, Taggart DP. Systematic review of therapies for stable coronary artery disease in diabetic patients. The Annals of Thoracic Surgery. 2015;**100**(6):2383-2397. DOI: 10.1016/j.athoracsur.2015.07.005 Epub 2015 Oct. 31

[38] Koskinas KC, Siontis GC, Piccolo R, et al. Impact of diabetic status on outcomes after revascularization with drug-eluting stents in relation to coronary artery disease complexity: Patient-level pooled analysis of 6081 patients. Circulation. Cardiovascular Interventions. 2016;**9**(2):e003255. DOI: 10.1161/CIRCINTERVENTIONS.115.003255

[39] Sumin AN, Bezdenezhnykh NA, Bezdenezhnyh AV, et al. Risk factors major cardiovascular events in the long term coronary artery bypass grafting in patients with coronary heart disease in the presence of type 2 diabetes (Russian). Russian Journal of Cardiology. 2015;**6**(122):30-37

[40] Gao L, Park SJ, Jang Y, Lee S, et al. Comparison of neoatherosclerosis and neovascularization between patients with and without diabetes: An optical coherence tomography study. JACC. Cardiovascular Interventions. 2015;**8**(8):1044-1052. DOI: 10.1016/j.jcin.2015.02.020

[41] Sumin AN, Bezdenezhnyh NA, Ivanov SV, et al. Factors associated with in-hospital mortality in coronary bypass surgery in patients with coronary artery disease combined with type 2 diabetes. (Russian). Diabetes Mellitus.2014;**4**:25-34

[42] Koochemeshki V, Salmanzadeh HR, Sayyadi H, et al. The effect of diabetes mellitus on short term mortality and morbidity after isolated coronary artery bypass grafting surgery. International Cardiovascular Research Journal. 2013;**7**(2):41-45

[43] Pang PY, Lim YP, Ong KK, et al. 2015 young surgeon's award winner: Long-term prognosis in patients with diabetes mellitus after coronary artery bypass grafting: A propensity-matched study. Annals of the Academy of Medicine, Singapore. 2016;**45**(3):83-90

[44] Lontchi-Yimagou E, Sobngwi E, Matsha TE, et al. Diabetes mellitus and inflammation. Current Diabetes Reports. 2013;**13**:435-444

[45] Tavlueva EV, Yarkovskaya AP, Barbarash OL. The relationship of diabetes with pro-inflammatory status in STEMI females and males. Complex Issues of Cardiovascular Diseases. 2014;**1**:42-46. DOI: 10.17802/2306-1278-2014-1

[46] Ujueta F, Weiss EN, Sedlis SP, et al. Glycemic control in coronary revascularization. Current Treatment Options in Cardiovascular Medicine. 2016;**18**(2):12. DOI: 10.1007/s11936-015-0434-6

[47] Chen PC, Chua SK, Hung HF, et al. Admission hyperglycemia predicts poorer short- and long-term outcomes after primary percutaneous coronary intervention for ST-elevation myocardial infarction. Journal of Diabetes Investigation. 2014;**5**:80-86. DOI: 10.1111/jdi.12113

[48] Trubnikova OA, Mamontova AS, Maleva OV, et al. Predictors of persistant post-operation cognitive dysfunction in 2 type diabetes patients after coronary bypass grafting (Russian). Russian Journal of Cardiology. 2016;**2**:12-18. DOI: 10.15829/1560-4071-2016-2-12-18

[49] Bruce DG. Type 2 diabetes and cognitive function: Many questions, few answers. Lancet Neurology. 2015;**14**(3):241-242. DOI: 10.1016/S1474-4422(14)70299-6

[50] Sathya B, Davis R, Taveira T, et al. Intensity of perioperative glycemic control and postoperative outcomes in patients with diabetes: A meta-analysis. Diabetes Research and Clinical Practice. 2013;**102**(1):8-15. DOI: 10.1016/j.diabres.2013.05.003

[51] Masoumi G, Frasatkhish R, Bigdelian H, et al. Insulin infusion on postoperative complications of coronary artery bypass graft in patients with diabetes mellitus. Research in Cardiovascular Medicine. 2014;**3**(2):e17861. DOI: 10.5812/cardiovascmed.17861

[52] Pezzella T, Holmes SD, Pritchard G, et al. Impact of perioperative glycemic control strategy on patient survival after coronary bypass surgery. The Annals of Thoracic Surgery. 2014;**98**:1281-1285. DOI: 10.1016/j.athoracsur.2014.05.067

[53] Umpierrez G, Cardona S, Pasquel F, et al. Randomized controlled trial of intensive versus conservative glucose control in patients undergoing coronary artery bypass graft surgery: GLUCO-CABG trial. Diabetes Care. 2015;**38**(9):1665-1672. DOI: 10.2337/dc15-0303

[54] Fox CS, Golden SH, Anderson C, et al. Update on prevention of cardiovascular disease in adults with type 2 diabetes mellitus in light of recent evidence: A scientific statement from the American Heart Association and the American Diabetes Association. Diabetes Care. 2015;**38**(9):1777-1803. DOI: 10.2337/dci15-0012

[55] Skyler JS, Bergenstal R, Bonow RO, et al. American Diabetes Association, American College of Cardiology Foundation, American Heart Association. Intensive glycemic control and the prevention of cardiovascular events: Implications of the ACCORD, ADVANCE, and VA Diabetes Trials: A position statement of the American Diabetes Association and a Scientific Statement of the American College of Cardiology Foundation and the American Heart Association. Journal of the American College of Cardiology. 2009;**53**(3):298-304. DOI: 10.1161/CIRCULATIONAHA.108.191305

[56] Pankov V. Clinical aspects of hypoglycemia as a risk factor for cardiovascular complications in type 2 diabetes. International Journal of Endocrinology. 2011;**5**(37): [Russian]

[57] Tennyson C, Lee R, Attia R, et al. Is there a role for HbA1c in predicting mortality and morbidity outcomes after coronary artery bypass graft surgery? Interactive Cardiovascular and Thoracic Surgery. 2013;**17**(6):1000-1008. DOI: 10.1093/icvts/ivt351

[58] Kinoshita T, Asai T, Suzuki T, et al. Preoperative hemoglobin A1c predicts atrial fibrillation after off-pump coronary bypass surgery. European Journal of Cardio-Thoracic Surgery. 2012;**41**(1):102-107. DOI: 10.1016/j.ejcts.2011.04.011

[59] Sumin AN, Bezdenezhnyh NA, Bezdenezhnyh AV, Ivanov SV, Barbarash OL. Factors associated with immediate results of coronary artery bypass grafting in patients with ischemic heart disease in the presence of type 2 diabetes. Kardiologiia. 2016;**10**:13-21. DOI: 10.18565/cardio.2016.10.13-21

[60] Schernthaner G. Diabetes and cardiovascular disease: Is intensive glucose control beneficial or deadly? Lessons from aCCORD, aDVaNCE, VaDT, UKPDS, PROactive, and NICE-SUGaR. Wiener Medizinische Wochenschrift (1946). 2010;**160**:8-19. DOI: 10.1007/s10354-010-0748-7

[61] Gerstein HC, Miller ME, Byington RP, et al. Action to control cardiovascular risk in diabetes study group. Effects of intensive glucose lowering in type 2 diabetes. The New England Journal of Medicine. 2008;**358**:2545-2559. DOI: 10.1056/NEJMoa0802743

[62] Patel A, MacMahon S, Chalmers J, et al., ADVANCE Collaborative Group. Intensive blood glucose control and vascular outcomes in patients with type 2 diabetes. The New England Journal of Medicine. 2008;**358**:2560-2572. DOI: 10.1056/NEJMicm066227

[63] Duckworth W, Abraira C, Moritz T, et al. Intensive glucose control and complications in American veterans with type 2 diabetes. The New England Journal of Medicine. 2009;**360**:129-139. DOI: 10.1056/NEJMoa0808431

[64] Inzucchi SE, Bergenstal RM, Buse JB, et al. Management of hyperglycemia in type 2 diabetes, 2015. Update to a position statement of the American Diabetes Association and the European Association for the Study of Diabetes. Diabetes Care. 2015;**38**:140-149. DOI: 10.2337/dc14-2441

[65] Hoogwerf BJ. Perioperative management of diabetes mellitus: How should we act on the limited evidence? Cleveland Clinic Journal of Medicine. 2006;**73**:95-99

[66] Shah B, Berger JS, Amoroso NS, et al. Periprocedural glycemic control in patients with diabetes mellitus undergoing coronary angiography with possible percutaneous coronary intervention. The American Journal of Cardiology. 2014;**113**:1474-1480. DOI: 10.1016/j.amjcard.2014.01.428

[67] Ike A, Shirai K, Nishikawa H, et al. Associations between different types of hypoglycemic agents and the clinical outcome of percutaneous coronary intervention in diabetic patients—From the FU-Registry. Journal of Cardiology. 2015;**65**:390-396. DOI: 10.1016/j.jjcc.2014.06.012

[68] Dangas GD, Farkouh ME, Sleeper LA, et al. Long-term outcome of PCI versus CABG in insulin and non-insulin-treated diabetic patients: Results from the FREEDOM trial. Journal of the American College of Cardiology. 2014;**64**:1189-1197. DOI: 10.1016/j.jacc.2014.06.1182

[69] Platoshkin NE, Kanus II. Clinical guidelines and evidence-based medicine position on the issue of perioperative management of patients with diabetes mellitus. Health and Environmental Problems. 2012;**3**(33):35-39

[70] Baradari AG, Zeydi AE, Aarabi M, et al. Metformin as an adjunct to insulin for glycemic control in patients with type 2 diabetes after CABG surgery: A randomized double blind clinical trial. Pakistan Journal of Biological Sciences. 2011;**14**(23):1047-1054

[71] Messaoudi SE, Nederlof R, Zuurbier CJ, et al. Effect of metformin pretreatment on myocardial injury during coronary artery bypass surgery in patients without diabetes (MetCAB): A double-blind, randomised controlled trial. The Lancet Diabetes and Endocrinology. 2015;**3**(8):615-623. DOI: 10.1016/S2213-8587(15)00121-7

[72] Li J, JP X, Zhao XZ, et al. Protective effect of metformin on myocardial injury in metabolic syndrome patients following percutaneous coronary intervention. Cardiology. 2014;**127**(2):133-139. DOI: 10.1159/000355574

[73] Ali MK, Bullard KM, Saaddine JB, et al. Achievement of goals in U.S. diabetes care, 1999-2010. The New England Journal of Medicine. 2013;**368**:1613-1624. DOI: 10.1056/NEJMsa1213829

[74] Moutzouri E, Tellis CC, Rousouli K, et al. Effect of simvastatin or its combination with ezetimibe on Toll-like receptor expression and lipopolysaccharide-induced cytokine production in monocytes of hypercholesterolemic patients. Atherosclerosis. 2012;**225**:381-387. DOI: 10.1016/j.atherosclerosis.2012.08.037

[75] Sattar NA, Ginsberg H, Ray K, et al. The use of statins in people at risk of developing diabetes mellitus: Evidence and guidance for clinical practice. Atherosclerosis. Supplements. 2014;**15**:1-15. DOI: 10.1016/j.atherosclerosissup.2014.04.001

[76] Stone NJ, Robinson JG, Lichtenstein AH, et al. 2013 ACC/AHA guideline on the treatment of blood cholesterol to reduce atherosclerotic cardiovascular risk in adults: A report of the American College of Cardiology/American Heart Association Task Force on Practice Guidelines. Circulation. 2014;**129**(25S2):1-45. DOI: 10.1161/01.cir.0000437738.63853.7a

[77] Miura M, Yamasaki M, Uemura Y, et al. Effect of statin treatment and low-density lipoprotein-cholesterol on short-term mortality in acute myocardial infarction patients undergoing primary percutaneous coronary intervention—Multicenter registry from Tokyo CCU Network Database. Circulation Journal. 2016;**80**(2):461-468. DOI: 10.1253/circj.CJ-15-0889

[78] Venkatesan S, Okoli GN, Mozid AM, et al. Effects of five preoperative cardiovascular drugs on mortality after coronary artery bypass surgery: A retrospective analysis of an observational study of 16,192 patients. European Journal of Anaesthesiology. 2016;**33**(1):49-57. DOI: 10.1097/EJA.0000000000000340

Chapter 5

Coronary Artery Bypass and Stroke: Incidence, Etiology, Pathogenesis, and Surgical Strategies to Prevent Neurological Complications

Marco Gennari, Gianluca Polvani,
Tommaso Generali, Sabrina Manganiello,
Gabriella Ricciardi and Marco Agrifoglio

Additional information is available at the end of the chapter

http://dx.doi.org/10.5772/intechopen.72389

Abstract

Current data suggest that cardiac bypass surgery is the single largest cause of iatrogenic stroke. Among the strategies to decrease or eliminate aortic manipulation, there is the use of off-pump coronary artery bypass grafting (CABG) through an aortic "no touch" technique, which reduces significantly the stroke rate. However, this off-pump aortic "no touch" technique is not always applicable, and, when saphenous vein and/or free arterial aortocoronary grafts are used, there is still risk of neurological injury due to tangential aortic clamp applied during the proximal anastomosis sewing. We aim to analyze the current incidence, etiology, and physiopathology of the neurological complications after coronary artery bypass surgery. We describe the methods and techniques that provide reduction in the occurrence of neurological complications. CABG with multiple clamp technique failed to find a better outcome in terms of neuropsychological deficit in the OPCABG group. By the way, patients undergoing CABG with single clamping seems to have better outcomes, suggesting that the cross-clamping technique used and minimal aortic manipulation could have had a role in reducing neurocognitive impairment. Moreover, surprisingly, CPB seemed to be a neuroprotective factor, and this aspect could be linked to the mild hypothermia used during on-pump surgery.

Keywords: coronary artery bypass, stroke, cardiac surgery, aortic cross clamp, neurologic impairment

1. Introduction

In 1978 the World Health Organization defined a stroke as a focal or global neurologic deficit due to cerebrovascular cause that persists beyond 24 hours or is interrupted by death within 24 hours [1].

Strokes are classified by etiology into **ischemic strokes** (85%) and **hemorrhagic strokes** (15%). Ischemic strokes result from a critical reduction in blood flow and are categorized as embolic, thrombotic, hemodynamic, or hypotensive [2].

Cerebrovascular accidents (CVAs) remain one of the most common complications after surgical myocardial revascularization despite the increased quality of treatment. Cerebral injuries are associated with substantial increases in mortality, morbidity, length of hospitalization, and an impaired quality of life [3].

Ischemic stroke occurs in 1.5–5.2% of patients. Percentage varies across studies and depends on study design, patient risk profile, operative techniques, and the length of study follow-up. Although advances in surgical and medical management have occurred across the last 10 years, the risk of stroke after coronary artery bypass grafting (CABG) has not significantly declined likely because of the progressive aging of the CABG population [4].

The etiology of postoperative stroke is multifactorial. Previous studies showed that the risk factors for postoperative stroke following CABG include age, low left ventricular ejection fraction, unstable angina, atherosclerosis of the ascending aorta, chronic renal failure, chronic obstructive pulmonary disease, calcified aorta, a history of previous stroke, carotid stenosis, duration of cardiopulmonary bypass, peripheral vascular disease, smoke, and diabetes mellitus. The age seems the most important risk factor for postoperative stroke, followed by palpable calcification in the ascending aorta and arch [5, 6].

1.1. Epidemiology

The prevalence of stroke after surgery varies according to the different types of surgery and patient comorbidities. A postoperative stroke is reported to occur in 0.08–0.7% of patients after general surgery, in 0.8–3% after peripheral vascular surgery, in 4.8% after head and neck surgery, in 2–3% after carotid endarterectomy, in 8.7% after aortic repair, and in 5.7% after cardiac surgery. Furthermore, patients with advanced age, previous stroke or transient ischemic attack (TIA), or postoperative atrial fibrillation are at increased risk for postoperative strokes [7, 8].

Most postoperative strokes do not occur immediately after surgery; there is usually a symptom-free interval before ischemia becomes apparent. In a recent retrospective study, only 8% of strokes appeared in the postanesthesia care unit. Approximately 45% of occurrences are identified within the first day after surgery [9].

The incidence of early stroke within 30 days of the myocardial surgery revascularization is reported to be 2–4%. Other studies indicated that the rate of postoperative stroke in octogenarians ranged from 2 to 9% [10].

Recent studies using sensitive brain magnetic resonance imaging (MRI) with diffusion-weighted imaging report that 45% of patients who have undergone cardiac surgery have new ischemic brain lesions that are often clinically undetected. For this reason, the prevalence of stroke can be higher than documented [11, 12].

2. Incidence and etiology of neurological events after cardiac surgery

2.1. Cerebral embolism

It is possible to divide emboli into two categories: microemboli and macroemboli according to size (200 μm or greater). This distinction reflects different clinical manifestations: a single macroembolus can result in hemiplegia; instead, a microembolus is unlikely to have a noticeable effect except when these emboli are numerous. Macroemboli are unlikely to arise from the extracorporeal circuit but rather from surgical manipulation of the heart and the aorta. There are other categories: gaseous, biologic, inorganic, etc [13].

Gaseous emboli are usually derived from air or anesthetic gas (such as nitrous oxide). These emboli are introduced into the left side of the heart (during aorta or mitral valve replacement) or into the aorta (from the bypass circuit). The superiority of membrane oxygenators compared with bubble oxygenators in reducing cardiopulmonary bypass (CPB)-generated embolism has been demonstrated by ultrasound and retinal angiography [14].

Inorganic embolism which can arise from embolization of fragments of polyvinyl chloride tubing exposed to roller pump has been described.

Biologic aggregates include thrombus, platelets, and fat. Thrombus can arise from the left appendage, the left ventricular aneurysm, or from the CPB circuit. Heparin may contribute to create fat embolism by stimulating endothelial lipoprotein lipase. It seems that the principal sources of cholesterol embolism are large vessels of atherosclerotic plaques.

2.2. Cerebral hypoperfusion

Although a postoperative stroke is most often embolic in origin, an association between intraoperative hypotension and the occurrence of a postoperative stroke is often assumed.

Some authors identified the watershed infarcts; these are areas of the brain that are between non-anastomosing arterial vessels and arteries. They are termed watershed or border-zone areas. They are critically dependent on adequate perfusion pressure in the border-zone vessels. A reduction in perfusion below a critical value will result in ischemia because of inadequate collateral circulation. Infarction of watershed areas has been regarded as the hallmark of hemodynamic strokes. There are two major watershed regions. The cortical watershed areas are between the cortical branches of the anterior, middle, and posterior cerebral arteries. The internal or subcortical watershed is located in the white matter along and slightly above the lateral ventricles between the deep (lenticulostriate) and the cortical branches of the middle cerebral artery and the anterior cerebral arteries. There is much controversy about the relative contribution of low-flow pathophysiology. For example, it is hard to determine whether a local low-flow state due to hypoperfusion results in platelet microemboli or whether platelet microemboli result in local hypoperfusion. Irrespective of the sequence, there is a synergistic interaction [15, 16].

Intraoperative hypotension is a common event during surgery. Bijker et al. reviewed four major anesthesia journals for their definitions of hypotension. Almost 50 different definitions were found utilizing systolic pressure and/or mean pressure either as an absolute or as a percentage of the baseline value. Diastolic pressure was never used. The most frequent definitions were as follows [17, 18]:

1. A 20% decrease in systolic pressure from the baseline value.
2. A combination of systolic pressures below 100 mmHg or greater than 30% decrease from the baseline value.
3. A systolic pressure below 80 mmHg. A definition of "baseline" was provided in only 50% of the manuscripts but was most frequently the blood pressure immediately before induction of anesthesia.

The majority of the articles stated how frequently blood pressure was measured, but only 10% of the articles specified a minimum duration for which reduced blood pressure would constitute hypotension.

Furthermore, it is possible to found a congenital variation of the circle of Willis. A persistent complete fetal-type posterior circulation results in the complete separation of the posterior and anterior circulations and occurs in 1–4% of the population. Development of collaterals usually occurs slowly, although hypoplastic vessels may have the capacity to be more acutely dilated. The contribution of the abnormalities to perioperative stroke is unknown, although, as shown in a recent case report, they may be an important factor for some patients [19, 20].

2.3. Atherosclerosis of the aorta

Aortic atherosclerosis is characterized by the formation of intimal plaques with the usual morphologic features of atherosclerosis, including cellular proliferation, lipid accumulation, inflammation, necrosis, fibrosis, and calcifications. Ulceration of these plaques can result in embolization of plaque elements or thrombus formation, which can lead to neurologic deficit, stroke, and death. Cardiac surgery usually involves manipulation of the ascending aorta by arterial cannulation and cross clamping. All of which can increase the risk of embolization of atherosclerotic material to the brain. The prevalence of atherosclerotic disease in the ascending aorta varies across studies, depending on the patient population, the criteria used to define the disease, and the diagnostic tool implemented to detect the disease. This type of disease has significantly increased in recent years, likely due to better diagnostic methods and an increasing population of elderly. Peripheral vascular disease, age, hypertension, and diabetes have been reported to be independent predictors of atherosclerotic disease of the ascending aorta [21].

The magnitude of this problem was well illustrated in a large prospective study by Roach et al. involving 24 centers. They reported a 3.1% incidence of type 1 neurologic injury (focal injury or stupor or coma at discharge) after CABG. Affected patients had a higher in-hospital mortality rate than patients without neurologic complications (21% vs. 2%), as well as a longer hospital stay (25 days vs. 10 days). Predictors of type I outcomes were palpable proximal aortic atherosclerosis, a history of neurologic disease, and older age. A high correlation between atherosclerosis of the ascending aorta and atheroembolism during CABG surgery has been established by several studies. Observational studies have shown, for example, that

http://dx.doi.org/10.5772/intechopen.72389

atherosclerosis of the ascending aorta detected at the time of surgery is an independent risk factor for stroke. A previous study documented that the presence of atherosclerosis alone in this region in patient undergoing cardiac surgery increased the risk of early postoperative stroke from 1.8 to 8.7%. It is widely postulated that the proximate cause of atheroembolism is disruption of the atheroma during surgical manipulations such as for aortic cannulation, aortic cross clamping, or proximal coronary artery anastomosis. These interventions are associated with increases in Doppler-detected cerebral embolic signals, but the composition of these emboli cannot be determined. Disruption of atherosclerotic lesions was verified in a study of 472 patients who underwent epiaortic ultrasound before and after CPB, with new mobile lesions of the ascending aorta identified in 10 (3.4%) of patients after surgery at sites of aortic clamping or cannulation and stroke occurring in 3 of these 10 patients. A smaller study by Ribakove et al. revealed a similar rate of stroke (3 out of 10) in patients with identified mobile lesions (31). Swaminathan et al. demonstrated the potential of atheroma disruption due to the "sandblasting" effect of CPB at the site of the aortic cannula [22, 23].

Injury involving atherosclerotic lesions not only can result in emboli during surgery but may also expose lipid-laden, prothrombotic material that could promote thrombus formation postoperatively after heparin neutralization. Finally, atherosclerosis of the ascending aorta identifies patients likely to have severe atherosclerosis of cerebral arteries who are prone to cerebral injury from hypoperfusion. For this reason, avoidance of significant hypotension during and after surgery may be prudent to avoid neurologic injury [24, 25].

2.4. Atrial fibrillation

Atrial fibrillation (AF) is the most common sustained arrhythmia encountered in clinical practice. Its prevalence increases with age, affecting approximately 1% of the total population and 8% of individuals over 80 years old. The incidence of postoperative AF following coronary artery bypass grafting (CABG) surgery is high and ranges between 20 and 40% of patients. It increases the length of hospital stay and hospital costs and is associated with increased morbidity and mortality including postoperative stroke, as well as in-hospital and 6-month mortality. Postoperative AF typically develops within the first week post surgery, at a median time of 2 days after the operation. It generally resolves within 24–48 hours, and most patients are discharged in sinus rhythm. Several factors have been found to predict the risk of postoperative AF following CABG, including enlarged left atrial size and prolonged hospitalization post surgery [26].

In medical patients with chronic or recurrent AF, the cause and effect relationship between the arrhythmia and the cerebrovascular event has been unquestionably proven [27].

Lahtinen and colleagues from Finland analyzed data of 52 stroke patients after CABG operation and found that in 19 patients (36%) the first AF episode preceded the development of stroke by a mean of 21.3 hours (average, 2.5 AF episodes before stroke). The stroke was attributed to calcification in the ascending aorta in 13 patients (25%), and 16 patients (31%) had greater than 70% internal carotid artery stenosis [28].

The pathophysiology of postoperative AF is not completely understood. Apart from obvious comorbid conditions such as valvular heart disease, atrial enlargement, congestive heart failure, and history of preoperative atrial arrhythmias, several other risk factors predispose cardiac surgical patients for postoperative AF. Advanced age is the strongest, followed by systemic hypertension, left ventricular hypertrophy, peripheral vascular disease, and chronic lung disease. Longer cardiopulmonary bypass time and aortic cross-clamping time have been shown to be associated with increased incidence of postoperative AF. Postoperative pericardial fluid collection and pericarditis have also been associated with atrial arrhythmias [29].

2.5. Genetic predisposition

It has been suggested that genetic predisposition might explain the marked variability in individual susceptibility for cerebral injury from cardiac surgery despite similar risk. Tardiff was the first to show a relationship between the risk of postoperative neurocognitive dysfunction and the presence of the apolipoprotein E ε4 allele. The apolipoprotein E (APOE) ε4 genotype is a plausible candidate gene since it has been shown to increase risk for Alzheimer's disease and cognitive decline after cerebral injury. Other investigators have examined for a relationship between polymorphisms of genes involved in pathways regulating coagulation, cell adhesion, and inflammation with perioperative cerebral injury [30].

The C-reactive protein minor allele 1059G/C SNP and the P-selectin allele SELP 1087G/A allele were further found to be associated with decline in cognition 6 weeks after CABG surgery.

Grocott et al. documented that the presence of at least one minor allele at each of the two loci (CRP, 3_UTR 1846C/T; IL-6, 74G/C) is a risk factor for stroke, increasing risk more than threefold (60). The observation that the interaction of these two inflammatory SNPs contributes to perioperative stroke suggests that inflammatory pathways may be important mechanistic factors in either initiating or otherwise modulating stroke after cardiac surgery. This interpretation is consistent with the current knowledge regarding CPB initiating and IL-6 mediating a robust inflammatory response. This finding is also consistent with the view that inflammation plays an important role in the etiology of stroke in the general population [31].

2.6. Carotid stenosis

Carotid artery atherosclerosis often accompanies significant coronary atherosclerotic lesions. Hypoperfusion arising from a severely stenotic carotid artery or embolization from an ulcerated plaque, calcific debris from a diseased valve, and introduction of air during the procedure are important mechanisms. The risk of stroke in patients with carotid artery disease after CABG has been estimated 1.8% in patients with stenosis <50%, 3.2% in patients with stenosis between 50 and 99%, and 10% in patients with contralateral occlusion. It is thought that carotid intra-plaque hemorrhage can result in plaque destabilization and intimal ulceration, creating a nidus for thromboembolism. Intra-plaque hemorrhage detected by magnetic resonance imaging is associated with increase of ipsilateral stroke in symptomatic and asymptomatic nonsurgical patients. Impaired cerebral hemodynamic functional distal to carotid artery stenosis is another determinant of postoperative stroke. Maximally dilated vessels distal to carotid artery stenosis can no longer vasodilate in response to hemodynamic compromise. Therefore, perioperative reduction in blood pressure or cardiac output in this group of patients is hypnotized to lead to cerebral ischemia [32, 33].

3. Pathogenesis of neurological complications in conventional coronary artery bypass grafting (CABG)

3.1. Risk factors of stroke after myocardial revascularization

The risk factors of postoperative stroke can be divided into preoperative, intraoperative, and postoperative factors [34].

Preoperative factors include advanced age, atherosclerosis in the ascending aorta, unstable angina, hypertension, history of stroke, and redo surgery. Emergency surgery is performed for critical left main coronary artery disease (more or equal to 70% luminal narrowing with or without angina), or unstable cardiac conditions are also significant predictors of stroke after CABG procedure.

Intraoperative factors include the endurance of extracorporeal circulation and aorta clamping or operation type. Some reports demonstrate that the number of revascularized vessels (more or equal to three) is associated with a higher incidence of stroke after CABG procedure.

Finally, **postoperative factors** include atrial fibrillation, microembolism detachment, and hypotension.

The single most important risk factor for post-myocardial revascularization stroke is atrial fibrillation, newly onset or chronic. This arrhythmia occurs in up to 20% of patients following a STEMI and is associated with a significant increase in risk for an in-hospital stroke.

It is also well known that a high correlation exists between atherosclerosis of the ascending aorta and atheroembolism during CABG surgery, as several studies show.

In a prospective multicenter study including more than 2000 patients, atherosclerosis of the ascending aorta was the strongest independent predictor of stroke associated with CABG. In the study by Bergman et al., extensive atherosclerotic disease of the ascending aorta was associated with a 31% risk of postoperative stroke. The risk depends on the presence, location, and extent of disease, whenever the aorta is surgically manipulated.

Age > 75, black race, peripheral vascular disease, diabetes, renal impairment, hypertension, any frailty, and no aspirin therapy on discharge are also strong independent predictors of ischemic stroke [8]. In particular, age shows a strong correlation with stroke: for each 1 year increase in age, the odds of stroke increases by 12% [35].

In addition, the incidence of postoperative stroke in patients with a history of stroke is significantly higher than in patient with no previous history of stroke. Maybe, these data are due to associated older age and more complicated comorbidities of these patients.

3.2. Pathogenesis of stroke after myocardial revascularization

The two mechanisms responsible for stroke after CABG procedure are ischemia and hemorrhage. Some studies suggest that pan-vascular inflammation may also play a role, especially in the setting of acute coronary syndromes.

Ischemia can be due to embolic events (from cardiac chambers, aorta, or other peripheral arteries), thromboembolism of intra- or extracranial vessels, or systemic hypoperfusion. Hypoperfusion stroke arises from hemodynamic compromise distal to the carotid/cranial artery stenosis and has been associated with the patients' capacity for cerebral autoregulation [36].

Hemorrhage is instead associated with hypertension or reperfusion of infarcted area. The interaction between embolism and hypoperfusion is generally considered to be a major cause of postoperative stroke. Hypoperfusion may contribute to embolism retention. Several studies have found multiple emboli in the cortical watershed of patients who died after cardiac surgery. A recent study from Cao and co-workers suggests that unstable angina, LVEF <50%, and hypotension are risk factors of postoperative recurrent stroke. All of these factors decrease brain perfusion, leading to stroke.

Embolic ischemic stroke is generally caused by an embolus from the left atrium, as in atrial fibrillation, or from the left ventricle, as in recent AMI. Embolization of atheromatous debris from the aorta, instead, is likely to occur at the time of cannulation of the vessel to establish cardiopulmonary bypass, when the aortic clamp is applied or released or when proximal graft anastomoses are performed using side-biting clamp. Cerebral emboli often coexist with intraoperative hypoperfusion, which impairs the clearance of microemboli and may be responsible of bilateral watershed infarcts after CABG. Cerebral hypoperfusion may be exacerbated by the coexistence of carotid artery stenosis, which is another important risk factor for intraoperative stroke [37].

Thrombotic thromboembolism is related to the atherosclerotic disease of the intracranial vessels or hematologic pathologies. Thromboembolic strokes are most frequently caused by thrombus formation at the site of the ulcerated atherosclerotic plaque on the carotid/cranial arteries, although the aortic arch can also be a site of thrombus formation.

Neurological events after CABG are classified as:

- **Type 1**: in case of focal stroke, transient ischemic attack, or fatal brain damage.
- **Type 2**: in case of diffuse brain injury with disorientation and intellectual deterioration, which are normally reversible.

The stroke that occurs within the first 24 hours after the CABG is a potentially devastating complication. It is associated with the increased hospital mortality.

3.3. Risk stratification

Identification of vulnerable patients at increased risk of stroke before CABG is of paramount importance for the surgical decision-making approach and informed consent. As previously said, age, diabetes, hypertension, peripheral vascular disease, renal failure, left ventricular dysfunction, and nonelective surgery have consistently been reported as risk factors of perioperative stroke in patients undergoing CABG surgery. All these risk factors can be assessed before surgery. The combination of these variables has generated several risk stratification tools that can be implemented before surgery, to determine the individual probability of stroke in patients undergoing CABG [38].

In the Charlesworth score, generated from 33,000 consecutive patients undergoing isolated CABG, seven variables are integrated, including age, diabetes, left ventricular ejection fraction <40%, female gender, priority of surgery, renal dysfunction ,and peripheral vascular disease. In the simpler model generated by McKhann et al., only three variables are considered: age, hypertension, and history of stroke. More recently, Hornero et al. generated and validated a new risk model (Pack2 score), including priority of surgery, peripheral vascular disease, preoperative cardiac failure/left ventricular ejection fraction <40%, and chronic kidney failure. Interestingly, in patients with Pack2 score ≥ 2, off-pump CABG significantly reduced the risk of stroke compared with on-pump CABG, whereas no difference was apparent between the two strategies of revascularization in patients with Pack2 score < 2. Further studies should externally validate this score and assess whether it is useful in clinical practice to select the optimal strategy of revascularization between on-pump and off-pump CABG in high-risk patients.

However, these risk stratification tools share a major limitation in disregarding two important risk factors—atherosclerotic disease of the ascending aorta and pre-existing cerebrovascular disease. These factors should always be analyzed to make the optimal strategy of coronary revascularization within Heart Team environment.

Unfortunately, severe atherosclerosis of the ascending aorta is often an unexpected intraoperative finding during CABG, especially if preoperative risk stratification has not been accurate. It still represents a challenge for the surgeon, and sometimes the operative strategy must be changed at the time of surgery. The methods to diagnose severe atherosclerosis in the ascending aorta before surgery include computed tomography scanning, transesophageal echocardiography, or magnetic resonance imaging. Intraoperative ultrasonographic scanning of the aorta can also be used to find atherosclerotic changes in the entire ascending aorta. It is a rapid, safe, and sensitive method, and in some studies, it has been found to be more accurate than both transesophageal echocardiography and computed tomography in detecting atheromatous debris in the ascending aorta.

Assessment of the neurological risk profile of patients before CABG is another essential step to plan the surgery and predict the patients' risk for postoperative stroke. The neurological profile of the patient should be carefully characterized, seeking for a history of stroke, the presence of initial neurocognitive disorders, or the presence of pre-existing cerebrovascular disease. Recent studies have also suggested that detection of cerebral ischemia by magnetic resonance imaging before CABG is strongly associated with the risk of postoperative stroke. Searching for carotid artery disease with echo Doppler before CABG is also a safer and cheaper method of screening, especially in high-risk patients.

4. Off-pump coronary artery bypass (OPCAB) and "no touch technique" as strategies to reduce the neurological risk

CPB is still the most diffused technique used to perform CABG. Even if debate on the superiority of on-pump CABG over off-pump CABG (OPCABG) is still open, evidences of prospective studies like ROOBY trial showed better results in terms of cumulative 1-year events for myocardial infarction and revascularization procedures and better rate of venous graft patency at 1 year, along with better Fitz-Gibbon grade for on-pump CABG [39].

While other studies such as the SMART trial highlighted no significant differences between the two techniques in terms of mortality, myocardial infarction, stroke, and recurrent angina or readmission for cardiac or noncardiac events, on-pump CABG is still the gold standard procedure, and CPB is the most widely applied technique.

However, the use of CPB has been advocated to be related with a certain risk of neurocognitive sequelae linked with inflammatory response and microembolism [40].

On the other hand, cannulation itself, cross clamping, and, more widely, aortic manipulation have showed to be linked with neurocognitive impairment.

This point was also taken into consideration in ROOBY trial, where patient evaluation with neuropsychological testing was performed in every case in order to investigate memory, attention, and visuospatial skills. All the tests failed to find any clinically significant difference between the two groups, but a better scoring in the clock-drawing test was reported for the off-pump group.

This aspect was also investigated in other studies with no clear results. Remarkably, Hammon et al. prospectively analyzed 237 high-risk patients undergoing OPCABG vs. CABG with single clamp technique [41].

CABG with multiple clamp technique failed to find a better outcome in terms of neuropsychological deficit in the OPCABG group. By the way, patients undergoing CABG with single clamping had better outcome, suggesting that the cross clamping technique used and minimal aortic manipulation could have had a role in reducing neurocognitive impairment. Moreover, surprisingly, CPB seemed to be a neuroprotective factor, and this aspect could be linked to the mild hypothermia used during on-pump surgery [42].

In our study, the aim was to evaluate the acute rate of neurovascular outcome in two relatively homogeneous groups of patients, treated by the same senior surgeon in the same time frame. Neurological evaluation included clinical exam and CT scan. Five patients were found to have experienced ischemic stroke (2%) with no significant clinical sequelae, probably because of the limited interested cerebral area. However, no difference in the stroke rate between the SAC and DAC groups could be found. This is in contrast with other studies. Tsang et al. in 2003 randomized 268 patients either to single or multiple clamps with a higher rate of cerebrovascular accident in the multiple clamp group.

This fact should be taken into account if considering their results. In our study, patients were selected to be at low risk of cerebrovascular accident in order to have less confounding factors [43].

Gerriets et al. have also advocated the use of intra-aortic filter but failed to show a clinical significant benefit in their randomized trial.

Other parameters such as biochemical markers have been evaluated. Dar et al. showed that in a series of 50 patients randomized to single or multiple clamping CABG, S-100 protein levels

http://dx.doi.org/10.5772/intechopen.72389

were significantly higher in the second group; the troponin T levels were also evaluated with no significance. However, no clinically significant differences were found between the two groups.

In our cohort, none of the techniques used showed to be superior in terms of stroke incidence over the other. As each technique has its own surgical advantages and disadvantages (for instance, more space to perform proximal anastomosis in SAC and direct evaluation of graft's length in DAC), the surgeon should choose the technique with which he is more confident in order to have the best surgical result, as good outcome with very low complications rate can be achieved with both techniques. However, in selected patients, according to the literature, it can be rational to reduce aortic manipulation in the presence of aortic atheromas and to use mild hypothermia in order to have better cerebral protection, and SAC strategy could be preferred over DAC. OPCABG and the use of double mammary graft or Y configuration could be advocated in the case of porcelain aorta in order to avoid aortic manipulation [44].

An interesting aspect, as reported by Hammon et al., is that neuropsychological deficits, even if absent and even not radiologically detectable early after operation, can appear over a period of 6 months, suggesting that a closer neurological follow-up should be taken into consideration especially in high-risk patients to better estimate the real neurological outcome [45].

Regarding the so-called no touch technique, i.e., performing CABG without touching the aorta by anastomosing the grafts to the in situ left and/or right mammary arteries, the main concern is the technical feasibility and the need for adequate mammary arteries caliber and coronary arteries run-off, in order to adequately distribute the blood flow to the coronary bed [46].

5. Conclusion

In conclusion, incidence of stroke seems to be independent from cross-clamping technique, and, more generally, we could infer that the global rate of stroke after CABG is probably more influenced by the presence of subjacent risk factors as aortic atheromas, carotid stenosis, and peripheral vascular disease.

Author details

Marco Gennari[1]*, Gianluca Polvani[1,2], Tommaso Generali[3], Sabrina Manganiello[1], Gabriella Ricciardi[1] and Marco Agrifoglio[1,2]

*Address all correspondence to: marcogennari.md@gmail.com

1 Centro Cardiologico Monzino, IRCCS, Milan, Italy

2 Department of Cardiovascular Sciences and Community Health, University of Milan, Italy

3 San Donato Hospital, IRCCS, Italy

References

[1] Roach GW, Kanchuger M, Mangano CM, et al. Adverse cerebral outcomes after coronary bypass surgery: Multicenter study of Perioperative Ischemia Research Group and the Ischemia Research and Education Foundation investigators. The New England Journal of Medicine. 1996;**335**:1857-1863

[2] McKhann GM, Grega MA, Borowicz LM Jr, et al. Stroke and encephalopathy after cardiac surgery: An update. Stroke. 2006;**37**:562-571

[3] John R et al. Multicenter review of preoperative risk factors for stroke after coronary artery bypass grafting. The Annals of Thoracic Surgery. 2000;**69**:30-36

[4] D'Ancona G, Saez de Ibarra JI, Baillot R, Mathieu P, Doyle D, Metras J, et al. Determinants of stroke after coronary artery bypass grafting. European Journal of Cardio-Thoracic Surgery. 2003;**24**:552-556

[5] Filsoufi F, Rahmanian PB, Castillo JG, Bronster D, Adams DH. Incidence, topography, predictors and long term survival after stroke in patients undergoing coronary artery bypass grafting. The Annals of Thoracic Surgery. 2008;**85**:862-870

[6] Mashour GA, Shanks AM, Kheterpal S. Perioperative stroke and associated mortality after noncardiac, nonneurologic surgery. Anesthesiology. 2011;**114**:1289-1296

[7] Bateman BT, Schumacher HC, Wang S, Shaefi S, Berman MF. Perioperative acute ischemic stroke in noncardiac and nonvascular surgery: Incidence, risk factors, and outcomes. Anesthesiology. 2009;**110**:231-238

[8] Selim M. Perioperative stroke. The New England Journal of Medicine. 2007;**356**:706-713

[9] Kam PC, Calcroft RM. Peri-operative stroke in general surgical patients. Anaesthesia. 1997;**52**:879-883

[10] Hogue CW Jr, Palin CA, Aerosmith JE. Cardiopulmonary bypass management and neurologic outcomes: An evidence-based appraisal of current practices. Anesthesia and Analgesia. 2006;**103**:21

[11] Leary MC, Caplan L. Technology insight: Brain MRI and cardiac surgery-detection of postoperative brain ischemia. Nature Clinical Practice. Cardiovascular Medicine. 2007;**4**:379

[12] Padayachee TS, Parsons S, Thebold R, Linley J, Goslin RG, Deverall PB. The detection of microemboli in the middle cerebral artery during cardiopulmonary bypass: A transcranial Doppler ultrasound investigation using membrane and bubble oxygenators. The Annals of Thoracic Surgery. 1987;**44**:298-302

[13] Blauth C, Smith PL, Arnold JV, Jagoe JR, Wootton R, Taylor KM. Influence of oxygenator type on the incidence and extent of microembolic retinal ischemia during cardiopulmonary bypass. Assessment by digital image analysis. The Journal of Thoracic and Cardiovascular Surgery. 1990;**99**:61-69

[14] Blauth CJ, Cosgrove DM, Webb BW, et al. Atheroembolism from the ascending aorta. An emerging problem in cardiac surgery. The Journal of Thoracic and Cardiovascular Surgery. 1992;**103**:1104-1112

[15] Drummond JC, Lee RR, Howell JP Jr. Focal cerebral ischemia after surgery in the "beach chair" position: The role of a congenital variation of circle of Willis anatomy. Anesthesia and Analgesia. 2012;**114**:1301-1303

[16] Bijker JB, van Klei WA, Kappen TH, van Wolfswinkel L, Moons KG, Kalkman CJ. Incidence of intraoperative hypotension as a function of the chosen definition: Literature definitions applied to a retrospective cohort using automated data collection. Anesthesiology. 2007;**107**:213-220

[17] Davila-Roman VG, Barzilai B, Wareing TH, et al. Intraoperative ultrasonographic evaluation of the ascending aorta in 100 consecutive patients undergoing cardiac surgery. Circulation. 1991;**84**:III47-III53

[18] Katz ES, Tunick PA, Rusinek H, et al. Protruding aortic atheromas predict stroke in elderly patients undergoing cardiopulmonary bypass: Experience with intraoperative transesophageal echocardiography. Journal of the American College of Cardiology. 1992;**20**:70-77

[19] Bergman P, van der Linden J. Atherosclerosis of the ascending aorta as a major determinant of the outcome of cardiac surgery. Nature Clinical Practice. Cardiovascular Medicine. 2005;**2**:246-251

[20] Blauth CI. Macroemboli and microemboli during cardiopulmonary bypass. The Annals of Thoracic Surgery. 1995;**59**:1300-1303

[21] Dávila-Román VG, Murphy SF, Nickerson NJ, et al. Atherosclerosis of the ascending aorta is an independent predictor of long-term neurologic events and mortality. Journal of the American College of Cardiology. 1999;**33**:1308-1316

[22] Hogue CW, Murphy SF, Schechtman KB, et al. Risk factors for early or delayed stroke after cardiac surgery. Circulation. 1999;**100**:642

[23] Wareing TH, Davilla-Roman VG, Barzilia B. Management of the severely atherosclerotic ascending aorta during cardiac operations. The Journal of Thoracic and Cardiovascular Surgery. 1992;**103**:453

[24] Barbut D, Hinton RB, Szatrowski TP, et al. Cerebral emboli detected during bypass surgery are associated with clamp removal. Stroke. 1994;**25**:2398

[25] Stump DA, Rogers AT, Hammon JW, et al. Cerebral emboli and cognitive outcome after cardiac surgery. Journal of Cardiothoracic and Vascular Anesthesia. 1996;**10**:113

[26] Go AS, Hylek EM, Phillips KA, et al. Prevalence of diagnosed atrial fibrillation in adults: National implications for rhythm management and stroke prevention: The AnTicoagulation and Risk Factors in Atrial Fibrillation (ATRIA) Study. Journal of the American Medical Association. 2001;**285**:2370-2375

[27] Almassi GH, Schowalter T, Nicolosi AC, et al. Atrial fibrillation after cardiac surgery: A major morbid event? Annals of Surgery. 1997;**226**:501-511

[28] Mathew JP, Fontes ML, Tudor IC, et al. A multicenter risk index for atrial fibrillation after cardiac surgery. Journal of the American Medical Association. 2004;**291**:1720-1729

[29] Ahlsson AJ, Bodin L, Lundblad OH, et al. Postoperative atrial fibrillation is not correlated to C-reactive protein. The Annals of Thoracic Surgery. 2007;**83**:1332-1337

[30] Frye RL, Kronmal R, Schaff HV, Myers WO, Gersh BJ. Stroke in coronary artery bypass graft surgery: An analysis of the CASS experience. The participants in the Coronary Artery Surgery Study. International Journal of Cardiology. 1992;**36**:213-221

[31] Gardner TJ, Horneffer PJ, Manolio TA, et al. Stroke following coronary artery bypass grafting: A ten-year study. The Annals of Thoracic Surgery. 1985;**40**:574-581

[32] Angelini GD, Penny WJ, el-Ghamary F, et al. The incidence and significance of early pericardial effusion after open heart surgery. European Journal of Cardio-Thoracic Surgery. 1987;**1**:165-168

[33] Henderson AS, Easteal S, Jorm AF, et al. Apolipoprotein E allele epsilon 4, dementia, and cognitive decline in a population sample. Lancet. 1995;**346**:1387

[34] Charlesworth DC, Likosky DS, Marrin CAS, Maloney CT, Quinton HB, Morton JR, Leavitt BJ, Clough RA, O'Connor GT. Development and validation of a prediction model for strokes after coronary artery bypass grafting. The Annals of Thoracic Surgery. 2003;**76**:463-443

[35] Redmond M, Greene PS, Goldsborough MA, Cameron DE, Stuart RS, Sussman MS, Watkins L Jr, Laschinger JC, McKhan GM, Johnston MV, Baumgartner WA. Neurological injury in cardiac surgical patients with a history of stroke. The Annals of Thoracic Surgery. 1996;**61**:42-47

[36] Stamou SC, Hill PC, Dangas G, Pfister AJ, Boyce SW, Dullum MK, Bafi AS, Corso PJ. Stroke after coronary bypass: Incidence, predictors, and clinical outcome. Stroke. 2001; **32**:1508-1513

[37] Dutta M, Hanna E, Das P, Steinhubi SR. Incidence and prevention of ischemic stroke following myocardial infarction: Review of current literature. Cerebrovascular Disease. 2006;**22**:331-339

[38] Van der Linden J, Hadjinikolaou L, Bergman P, Lindblom D. Postoperative stroke in cardiac surgery is related to the location and extent of atherosclerotic disease in the ascending aorta. Journal of the American College of Cardiology. 2001;**38**:131-135

[39] Roach GW, Kanchuger M, Mangano CM, et al. Adverse cerebral outcomes after coronary bypass surgery. Multicenter Study of Perioperative Ischemia Research Group and the Ischemia Research and Education Foundation Investigators. New England Journal of Medicine. 1996;**335**:1857-1863

[40] Bergman P, van der Linden J. Atherosclerosis of the ascending aorta as a major determinant of the outcome of cardiac surgery. Nature Clinical Practice. Cardiovascular Medicine. 2005;**2**:246-251

[41] Lichtman JH, Krumolz HM, Wang Y, Radford M, Brass LM. Risk and predictors of stroke after myocardial infarction among the elderly. Results from co-operative cardiovascular project. Circulation. 2002;**105**:1082-1087

[42] AlWaqfi N, Ibraheem K, BaniHani M. Stroke after coronary artery surgery: Incidence and risk factors analysis. The Internet Journal of Cardiovascular Research. 2008;**7**(1)

[43] Cao et al. Risk factors for recurrent stroke after coronary artery bypass grafting. Journal of Cardiothoracic Surgery. 2011;**6**:157

[44] Grau AJ, Boddy AW, Dukovic DA, et al. Leukocyte count as an independent predictor of recurrent ischemic events. Stroke. 2004;**35**:1147-1152

[45] Schoof J, Lubahn W, Baeumer M, Kross R, Wallesch CW, Kozian A, Huth C, Goertler M. Impaired cerebral autoregulation distal to carotid stenosis occlusion is associated with increased risk of stroke at cardiac surgery with cardiopulmonary bypass. Journal of Thoracic and Cardiovascular Surgery. 2007;**134**:690-696

[46] Likosky DS, Marrin CAS, Caplan MR, Baribeu YR, Morton JR, Weintraumb MR, et al. Determination of etiologic mechanisms of stroke secondary to coronary artery bypass graft surgery. Stroke. 2003;**34**:28303-28304

Section 2

Management After Coronary Artery Bypass Surgery

Chapter 6

Arrhythmias Post Coronary Artery Bypass Surgery

Bandar Al-Ghamdi

Additional information is available at the end of the chapter

http://dx.doi.org/10.5772/intechopen.70423

Abstract

Arrhythmias are common after cardiac surgery such as coronary artery bypass grafting surgery. Although most of these arrhythmias are transient and have a benign course, it may represent a significant source of morbidity and mortality. Postoperative arrhythmias (POAs) include atrial tachyarrhythmias, ventricular arrhythmias, and bradyarrhythmias. The incidence of POAs has not changed despite improvements in anesthetic and surgical techniques. The tachyarrhythmias in the postoperative period include atrial fibrillation, atrial flutter, supraventricular tachycardia, and ventricular tachycardia. The clinical significance of each arrhythmia depends on several factors that include cardiac function, patient's comorbidities, arrhythmia duration, and ventricular response rate. Tachycardia with uncontrolled ventricular rates can cause diastolic and later on systolic dysfunction, reduce cardiac output, and result in hypotension or myocardial ischemia. In the other hand, bradyarrhythmias may have a remarkable influence on patients with systolic or diastolic ventricular dysfunction. Arrhythmia management starts preoperatively with optimizing the patient's condition and controlling patient's risk factors, intraoperatively with careful attention to hemodynamic changes during surgery and uses appropriate anesthesia, and postoperatively with correction of temporary and correctable predisposing factors, as well as specific therapy for the arrhythmia itself. The POAs treatment urgency and management options are determined by the clinical presentation of the arrhythmia.

Keywords: coronary artery bypass surgery, arrhythmias, atrial fibrillation, ventricular arrhythmias, bradyarrhythmias

1. Introduction

Arrhythmias are common after cardiac surgery such as coronary artery bypass grafting (CABG) surgery and represent a significant source of morbidity and mortality. Although most of these arrhythmias are transient and have a benign course, it may prolong intensive care and hospital stay, and in rare instances, it may lead to mortality. Postoperative arrhythmias (POAs) include atrial tachyarrhythmias (ATs) and to a lesser extent ventricular arrhythmias (VAs) and bradyarrhythmias [1]. The incidence of POAs has not changed despite improvements in anesthetic and surgical techniques, and evidence suggests that its incidence may be increasing [2].

The clinical significance of each arrhythmia depends on several factors that include underlying cardiac function, patient's comorbidities, arrhythmia duration, and ventricular response rate. So, POAs could be tolerated in some patients and a source of morbidity and mortality in others, depending on the interaction between these factors [1, 3]. Rapid ventricular rates with tachycardia can cause diastolic and later on systolic dysfunction, reduce cardiac output, and result in hypotension or myocardial ischemia [4, 5]. Bradydysrhythmias, particularly with the loss of atrial function, may have a remarkable influence on patients with systolic or diastolic ventricular dysfunction [6].

Arrhythmia management starts preoperatively with optimization of the patient's condition and controlling patient's risk factors. Intraoperatively, it includes careful attention to hemodynamic changes during surgery and uses appropriate anesthesia. Postoperatively, it includes correction of temporary and correctable predisposing factors, as well as specific therapy for the arrhythmia itself [7]. The POAs treatment urgency and management options are determined by the clinical presentation of the arrhythmia [7]. Self-terminating arrhythmias without overt cardiac disease often need no therapy. However, arrhythmias with hemodynamic instability, especially in patients with critical stress conditions like systemic infections or persistent pericardial effusion need urgent intervention to restore a stable clinical status [7].

The aim of this chapter is to review post-CABG arrhythmias pathophysiology and management.

2. Pathophysiology

The primary function of CABG is to reestablish perfusion to ischemic myocardium with utilizing autologous arteries and veins. This may be achieved by using different surgical techniques. The POAs pathophysiology, incidence, and clinical course may vary depending on the surgical techniques used. Initially, cardiac surgeries were performed on a beating heart, but with the development of cardiopulmonary bypass (CPB) machine and cardioplegia, most CABG surgeries were performed on a pump. However, interest in off-pump coronary artery bypass (OPCAB) surgery had revived in the 1990s [8]. Reported potential benefits of OPCAB include lower end-organ damage with less cerebrovascular accidents (CVA), fewer cognitive deficits, renal failure, less psychomotor defects, reduced systemic inflammation, and lower transfusion rates [9]. However, variable outcomes have been reported in studies comparing these strategies [9]. Minimally invasive surgery without use of CPB and through smaller incisions- and robotic-assisted approaches have also been developed [9]. This method is most often used for left internal mammary artery (LIMA) to left anterior descending artery (LAD) grafts. Additional benefits may also include reduced operative time, reduced recovery time, decreased the need for blood transfusion, less time under anesthesia, reduced duration of ICU stay, less pain, and an estimated 40% savings over conventional CABG [10].

The development of POAs is related to factors that influence the atrial and ventricular myocardium. These primarily include: a previous *anatomic substrate*, caused by degenerative changes typical of age and underlying disease, and *electrical substrate* derived from the perioperative processes that alter the membrane potentials, increase the dispersion of the refractory periods, and decrease the conduction velocity [11]. Inflammation and hyperadrenergic state appear to play a fundamental role in the development of postoperative tachyarrhythmias, favoring automatism [11]. Hypokalemia and hypomagnesemia characteristic of this period alter phase III of the membrane action potential, increasing the automatism, and slowing the conduction speed [11]. Atrial and ventricular ischemia due to hypoxemia is another contributing factor [11].

Several perioperative risk factors have been implicated in atrial and ventricular susceptibility to POAs, but their relative role is still uncertain. Risk factors for POAs may be classified into patient- and surgery-related factors [7].

2.1. Patient-related risk factors

Various patient-related risk factors have been described to cause POAs. These include:

2.1.1. Age

Increasing age is associated with age-related structural and electrophysiological changes that may lead to postoperative atrial tachyarrhythmias in the elderly. Old age has been demonstrated to be correlated with the development of POAs [2, 3, 12–14].

2.1.2. Underlying structural heart disease

Patients with underlying structural heart disease are at higher risk of developing POAs compared to patients with a normal heart. Structural heart disease in the atria and ventricles provides a substrate for arrhythmia via abnormal automaticity, triggered activity, or reentry. Cardiac surgery patients often have the substrate of atrial enlargement and elevation of atrial pressures may function as a substrate for atrial arrhythmias. It is well known that large atrial size and fibrosis supports propagation of atrial reentrant circuits and helps in maintaining atrial fibrillation (AF). Similarly, patients with ventricular dysfunction, ventricular dilation, or fibrosis are at higher risk of having ventricular arrhythmias [4]. Other important risk factors for POAs include previous history of arrhythmias (e.g., AF), cardiac surgery, and POAs. Also, severe right coronary artery stenosis [15], sinus nodal or atrioventricular nodal branch disease [13, 16, 17], and mitral valvular disease (particularly rheumatic mitral stenosis) have been reported as risk factors for POAs. The preoperative brain natriuretic peptide plasma concentration is another predictor of POAs [18].

2.1.3. Other comorbidities

Noncardiac comorbidities have been reported to increase the risk of POAs especially AF. These include obesity [19], previous stroke, and history of chronic obstructive pulmonary disease [20].

2.2. Surgery-related risk factors

Cardiac surgery may lead to POAs via multiple surgery-related mechanisms and risk factors that include:

2.2.1. Trauma and inflammation

Cardiac surgery provokes a vigorous inflammatory response due to a variety of metabolic, endocrine, and immune changes known as the "stress response," which has important clinical implications [21, 22] (**Figure 1**). Surgical trauma, blood loss or transfusion, hypothermia, and CPB are nonspecific activators of the inflammatory response [18, 19]. Surgical trauma may contribute to a higher degree of the inflammatory response compared to CPB [23]. These effects predispose to atrial and ventricular arrhythmias in the early postoperative period. Inflammatory mechanisms have been proposed for the development of postoperative AF (POAF) as its incidence peaks at early postoperative days. Inflammation may be related to the development of clinically aberrant or silent pericarditis. Unfortunately, clinical criteria, such as fever, pleuritic chest pain, pericardial rubs, and electrocardiogram changes correlate poorly with postoperative pericarditis and supraventricular arrhythmias [7]. However, patients with pericardial effusion in one study had a higher incidence of supraventricular arrhythmias (63% compared with 11% in patients without effusions) [24].

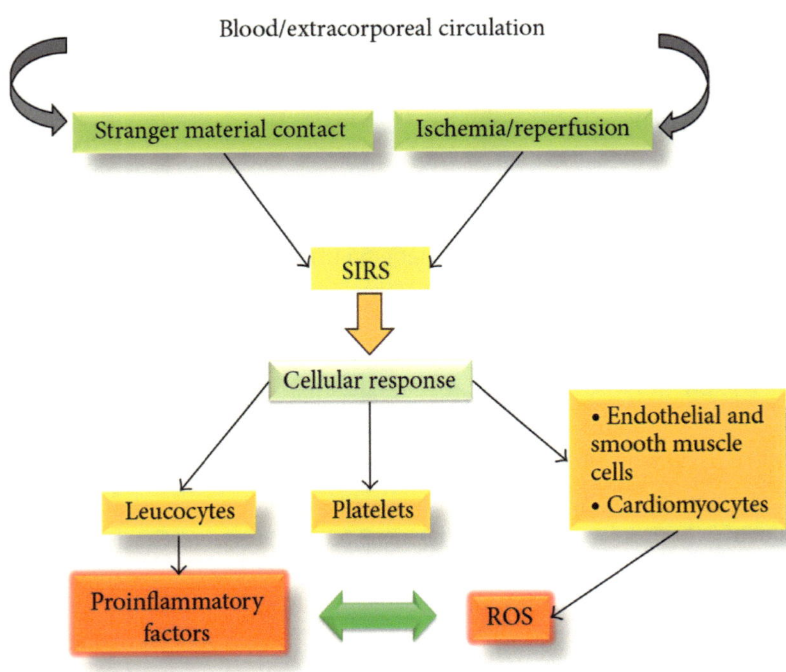

Figure 1. Pathophysiologic changes in response to cardiopulmonary bypass and the extracorporeal circulation. ROS, reactive oxygen species; SIRS, systemic inflammatory response syndrome (from Ref. [22]).

2.2.2. *Hemodynamic stress*

Atrial and ventricular hemodynamic changes during CABG predispose to POAs. The risk factors for POAs include atrial changes at the time of cardiac surgery, such as acute atrial trauma from cannulation, enlargement, hypertension, and ischemia [7]. Postoperative pulmonary edema and postoperative pleural effusion requiring thoracentesis have also been described as possible risk factors [25]. Hemodynamic changes might trigger focal arrhythmias [7]. It is possible that atrial stretch, hypertension, pressure and volume shifts, and heightened catecholamine states can trigger AF foci from the pulmonary veins [26].

2.2.3. *Ischemic injury*

The coronary blood flow is interrupted during CABG surgery and CPB, and the heart is put under circulatory arrest. This interruption of coronary blood flow causes ischemia-reperfusion injury that is exacerbated by adverse neutrophil-mediated myocardial inflammation and injury [27–29]. Atrial and ventricular ischemia or infarction triggers POAs [30]. Myocardial focal ischemia may occur due to endogenous or exogenous catecholamines, hypoxemia, hypercarbia, acid-base imbalances, drug effects, and mechanical factors. CPB, cross-clamp times, type of cardioplegia, and CABG surgical technique are also critical in determining ischemic injury. The incidence of AF has been demonstrated to be lower after OPCAB than conventional CABG. OPCAB is also associated with a lesser degree of inflammation [21].

2.2.4. *Perioperative drugs*

Beta-blocker withdrawal has been associated with an increased rate of postoperative supraventricular arrhythmias [31]. In contrary, some studies showed that preoperative digoxin use is a risk factor for POAs [2, 32], but not in the others [33]. Intravenous inotropic agents may be associated with POAs in some patients. The reported primary arrhythmias are sinus tachycardia (ST) and premature ventricular beats (PVCs), although other supraventricular (SVT) or ventricular arrhythmias (VT) have been reported. Clinically significant proarrhythmic effects with these agents appear to occur rarely. At conventional doses, intravenous inotropic agents are relatively safe concerning proarrhythmic effects. Inotropic agents increase sinoatrial node automaticity and decrease atrioventricular (AV) nodal conduction time [34, 35]. Dobutamine use has been reported to induce ventricular ectopic activity in 3–15% of patients [34]. Dopamine is more likely to be associated with a dose-related ST or AF [34]. Finally, short-term intravenous administration of the phosphodiesterase inhibitors amrinone and milrinone has been reported to cause PVCs and short runs of VT in up to 17% of patients [34]. Amiodarone and sotalol are useful and can be considered appropriate alternatives in high-risk patients [36]. Patients who need urgent CABG may benefit from intravenous and oral amiodarone combination in addition to beta-blockers. Although corticosteroids are associated with risk, it may be considered in selected CABG patients [36].

2.2.5. *Electrolytes disorders*

Hypokalemia leads to alteration of the electrophysiologic properties of cardiac myocytes with an increase in the action potential duration (increase in phase-3 depolarization), enhanced automaticity (increased slope of diastolic depolarization), and decreased conduction velocity [37]. These changes may provoke POAs [37]. Preoperative serum potassium levels of <3.5 mmol/L have a significant association with perioperative arrhythmias in patients undergoing elective CABG surgery [37].This association might be particularly evident in the atria, where changes in inward-rectifier potassium currents are supposed to act as profibrillatory mechanisms [38]. However, hypokalemia is more likely to be associated with VAs [38]. Moreover, it is worth noting that arrhythmogenesis is often multifactorial. Catecholamine release increases cellular potassium uptake and thus decreases serum potassium levels [39]. Serum potassium levels greater than 5.5 mmol/L appear to be associated with the development of POAF and atrial flutter (AFL) [37]. The role of magnesium remains controversial. The low serum magnesium levels—which is frequently seen after cardiac surgery—correlate with an increased incidence of POAs [7]. However, magnesium supplementation has produced conflicting results. Magnesium supplementation should be considered in all patients with hypomagnesemia [40–41].

2.2.6. Other factors

The human epicardial fat pads (FPs) contain parasympathetic ganglia [42]. There are two posterior FPs with the first one located in the superior vena caval-atrial junction and contains postganglionic fibers that lead to the sinoatrial (SA) node. The second FP is located at the pulmonary vein-left atrium and contains postganglionic fibers that lead to the atrioventricular (AV) node [43–45]. The anterior epicardial FP located in the aortopulmonary window that is routinely dissected and removed in CABG because it is located where the aortic cross-clamp is typically placed. Preservation of the human anterior epicardial FP during CABG decreases the incidence of POAF in one study [46], but not in another more recent study [47].

3. Postoperative atrial tachyarrhythmias (POATs)

3.1. Postoperative atrial fibrillation (POAF)

3.1.1. Epidemiology

AF is the most common complication seen after CABG surgery. The incidence of POAF is approximately 30% after isolated CABG, 40% after valve replacements or repair, and about 50% after combined CABG and valve surgeries [2, 48–51]. The incidence of POAF increases with older age [2, 52, 53].

3.1.2. Diagnosis

The diagnosis of POAF is confirmed based on the telemetry and 12-lead electrocardiogram (ECG) recordings with an abrupt change in heart rate and rhythm, and loss of P waves [16, 54]. Atrial electrograms obtained from temporary atrial epicardial pacing wires that are often routinely placed at the time of cardiac surgery can be helpful in confirming the diagnosis of AF, AFL, and other forms of supraventricular tachycardia (SVTs) [54].

3.1.3. Clinical course

POAF usually occurs within 2–4 days after cardiac surgery, with a peak incidence on the second postoperative day [12, 55]. In POAF patients without a prior history of atrial arrhythmias, AF is usually self-limited. About 15–30% of POAF convert to sinus rhythm within 2 h and up to 80% within 24 h [56, 57]. The mean duration of AF in one report was 11–12 h [57], and >90% of the patients were in sinus rhythm 6–8 weeks after surgery [57, 58]. In another study, only 2 out of 112 patients who had paroxysmal AF after CABG were still in AF at 6 weeks [59].

3.1.4. Prognosis

Although POAF is often self-limiting, its clinical effects depend on ventricular rate, ventricular function, arrhythmia duration, symptoms, hemodynamic stability, and risk of thromboembolism. [60]. POAF is associated with increased postoperative thromboembolic risk and stroke [25, 60–62]. In a series of 4507 patients, the incidence of stroke was significantly higher in those who developed POAF (3.3 versus 1.4%) [2]. Patient's underlying comorbidities, such as older age, previous cerebrovascular disease (CVA), the presence of a carotid bruit, peripheral vascular disease (PVD), and CPB time, have an important role in the development of in-hospital stroke [63–65]. In a review of 2972 patients undergoing CABG and/or valve surgery, POAF was associated with late onset stroke only if accompanied by a low cardiac output syndrome (3.9 versus 1.9%) [66]. Besides, POAF development is associated with a prolonged length of hospitalization [2, 25, 54]. The POAF is associated with an additional 2–4 days hospital stay after CABG surgery with an additional cost [54]. However, this effect seems to be less prominent with current cardiac surgical care [67]. Additionally, POAF may result in hemodynamic compromise [68], ventricular dysrhythmias [2], and iatrogenic complications associated with therapeutic interventions [53]. POAF may result in increased in-hospital and long-term mortality in a subset of patients [3, 60]. In a retrospective study of 6475 patients undergoing CABG at a single institution: 994 patients (15%) developed POAF. Higher in-hospital (7.4 versus 3.4%) and 4-year mortality (26 versus 13%) was noted in POAF patients but also with more comorbidities (i.e., older age, hypertension, and left ventricular hypertrophy) [60].

3.1.5. POAF management

The management of POAF should include the strategy for prevention and treatment of POAF when it develops. PAOF management starts with the optimization of medical comorbidities, if possible (e.g., hypoxia), and the correction of underlying electrolyte disturbances (e.g., potassium and magnesium abnormalities) [53]. POAF is treated similarly to AF in nonsurgical patients by rhythm control via pharmacological or electrical approach or heart rate control, and appropriate antithrombotic therapy.

3.1.5.1. Rhythm control versus heart rate control

In the atrial fibrillation follow-up investigation of rhythm management (AFFIRM) trial, the rate control versus rhythm control in nonsurgical patients with AF was studied and found that the use of rhythm control had no survival advantage, and it was associated with more frequent hospitalizations and adverse drug effects [69]. However, some studies involving patients with AF after cardiac surgery have suggested that rhythm control may offer advantages over rate control. This is still controversial and the evidence is inconclusive [11, 70–72].

Treatment strategies of POAF aim to reduce symptoms, limit adverse hemodynamic effects, decrease the length of hospital stay, prevent readmissions, and improve survival [73]. The rhythm control strategy has the advantage of a rapid conversion to sinus rhythm, which restores atrial activity, functional capacity, and might reduce thromboembolic. The rate control strategy has the advantage of avoiding the potential adverse effects of antiarrhythmic drugs and complications associated with cardioversion [73]. In a recent trial, there was no difference in hospital admissions during a 60-day follow-up, with randomizing POAF patients to either rhythm control therapy with amiodarone or rate control [73]. As a result, the main aim of rhythm control therapy in POAF patients should be to improve AF-related symptoms. In asymptomatic patients and those with acceptable symptoms, rate control or deferred cardioversion preceded by anticoagulation is a reasonable approach [73].

In the following paragraph, rate control and rhythm control options will be discussed briefly.

(A) Rate control strategy: the rate control may be achieved by using beta-blockers, nondihydropyridine calcium channel blockers, digoxin, or a combination of these medications. Beta-blocker agents are the drug of choice, particularly for ischemic heart disease patients, because of the increased adrenergic stress in the postoperative period [53, 73, 74]. However, beta-blockers might be poorly tolerated or relatively contraindicated in patients with known bronchial asthma or bronchospastic lung diseases, active congestive heart failure, or AV conduction block [53]. The nondihydropyridine calcium channel blocker agents represent an alternative AV nodal blocking agent. Digoxin is less effective when the adrenergic tone is as high as in the postoperative period, but it may be used in patients with congestive heart failure. Amiodarone is another agent that can be used as it has been reported to be effective in controlling heart rate. Also, intravenous amiodarone administration has been associated with improved hemodynamic status [75, 76]. For further information about drugs used in AF rate control see **Table 1**.

(B) Rhythm control: the rhythm control could be archived by using a direct current cardioversion (electrical cardioversion) or antiarrhythmic drugs (pharmacological cardioversion). Electrical cardioversion is indicated on an urgent basis in hemodynamically unstable patients, acute heart failure, or myocardial ischemia. Also, it may be used electively to restore sinus rhythm when a pharmacologic attempt has failed to resume a sinus rhythm [53]. Rhythm control with antiarrhythmic medications is preferred in symptomatic patients despite rate control trial, or when the control of ventricular response is hard to achieve. Amiodarone [77–79] or vernakalant [79, 80] have been efficient in converting POAF to sinus rhythm. Other antiarrhythmic medications that may be used include procainamide [80], ibutilide [81], and sotalol [82]. With ibutilide use, electrolyte imbalance should be corrected to avoid polymorphic ventricular tachycardia [82]. For further information about drugs used in AF rhythm control see **Table 2**.

3.1.5.2. Anticoagulation

POAF is associated with poor short- and long-term outcomes, including high rates of early and late stroke, and late mortality as mentioned earlier. However, the indication and timing of anticoagulation in POAF patients should take into consideration the risk of postoperative bleeding.

http://dx.doi.org/10.5772/intechopen.70423

Drug	Route of admintration and doses	Side effects sects	Remarks
Beta-blockers			
Atenolol	Oral 25–100 mg QD	Bradycardia, hypotension, fatigue, depression, negative inotropy, bronchospasm, AVB	Decrease dose if CrCl <35
Bisoprolol	Oral 2.5–10 mg QD	As above	Good choice for HF patients
Carvedilol	Oral 3.125–25 mg BID	As above	Good choice for HF patients
Esmolol	I.V. 500 mcg/kg bolus over 1 min, then 50–300 mcg/kg/min	As above	Only IV Higher rate of hypotension
Metoprolol tartrate	IV 2.5–5.0 mg bolus over 2 min; up to 3 doses Oral 25–100 mg BID	As above	
Metoprolol XL (succinate)	Oral 50–400 mg QD	As above	Good choice for HF patients
Nadolol	Oral 10 (usual initial adult dose 40 mg)–240 mg QD	As above	Dosage adjustments based on CrCl
Propranolol	IV 1 mg over 1 min, up to 3 doses at 2-min intervals Oral 10–40 mg up to 160–320 mg/day divided in BID to QID doses 80–160 to 320 mg QD (ER)	As above	
Calcium channel blockers			
Diltiazem	IV 0.25 mg/kg bolus over 5 min followed by 0.05–0.15 mg/kg/h continuous infusion Oral 30 mg TID/QID up to 480 mg/day 120–360 to 480 mg Q D (ER)	Bradycardia, hypotension, ankle swelling, exacerbation of HF, AVB	Do not use in HF Drug interaction via CYP3A4 including digoxin and warfarin
Verapamil	IV 5–10 mg (0.075–0.15 mg/kg) over bolus at least 2 min; may give an additional 10 mg (0.15 mg/kg) after 30 min if no response, then 0.005 mg/kg/min infusion Oral 80–120 mg TID up to 480 mg/day 180–480 mg QD or 240 BID (ER)	Bradycardia, AVB, hypotension, constipation, exacerbation of HF	As diltiazem
Others			
Digoxin	IV 0.25 mg IV with repeat dosing to a maximum of 1.5 mg over 24 h Oral 0.125–0.25 mg QD	Bradycardia, AVB, nausea, vomiting, visual disturbance	Narrow therapeutic window Adjust for renal failure Drug interactions via p-glycoprotein
Amiodarone	IV 150 mg over 10 min, followed by 1 mg/min continuous IV infusion for 6 h, then 0.5 mg/min continuous infusion for 18 h Oral 400–800 mg/day PO in divided doses for 2–4 weeks to a total load of up to 10 g, then 100–200 mg QD	Bradycardia, hypotension, AV block, QTc prolongation, phlebitis on chronic use: Ocular, pulmonary, hepatic, hematological, neurological complications	Monitor thyroid, liver and lung functions

AVB, atrioventricular block; CrCl, creatinine clearance; BID, twice daily; h, hour; ER, extended release; HF, heart failure; IV, intravenous; mg milligram; min, minute; QD, once daily; QID, 4 times a day; QTc, correct QT interval; TID, 3 times a day.

Table 1. Medications commonly used for atrial fibrillation **rate control** with its dosage and common possible side effects.

Drug	Usual doses	Side effects sects	Additional information
Vaughan Williams class IA			
Disopyramide	**Oral** IR 100–200 mg q 6 h ER 200–400 mg q 12 h	HF Prolonged QT interval Prostatism Glaucoma	Metabolized by CYP3A4: caution with inhibitors (e.g., verapamil, diltiazem, ketoconazole, macrolide antibiotics, protease inhibitors, grapefruit juice) and inducers (e.g., phenytoin, phenobarbital, rifampin) Avoid other QT interval prolonging drugs
Procainamide	**IV** 15–17 mg/kg infused at a rate of 20–30 mg/min or alternatively100 mg IV every 5 min, max. 1 g MD 1–4 mg/min	HF Prolonged QT interval May cause hypotension, myopathies, blood dyscrasias, and SLE-like syndrome	Drug of choice for WPW with AF Avoid other QT interval prolonging drugs Adjust for renal failure
Quinidine	**Oral** IR 200–300 mg q 6–8 h up to 600 mg q 6 h ER 324 mg–648 mg q 8–12 h	Prolonged QT interval Diarrhea Bradycardia, AV block, bundle-branch block, digitalis toxicity	Inhibits CYP2D6: ⇧ concentrations of metoprolol, tricyclic antidepressants, antipsychotics; ⇩ efficacy of codeine Inhibits P-glycoprotein:⇧ digoxin concentration
Vaughan Williams class IC			
Flecainide	**IV** 1.5–3 mg/kg over 10-20 min **Oral** LD 200 (wt < 70 kg)–300 mg (wt > 70 kg), MD 50–200 mg BID max. 400 mg/day	Sinus or AV node dysfunction HF CAD Atrial flutter Brugada syndrome Renal or liver disease May cause blurred vision	Metabolized by CYP2D6 (inhibitors include quinidine, fluoxetine, tricyclics; also genetically absent in 7–10% of population) and renal excretion (dual impairment can ⇧⇧ plasma concentration) Decrease dose if CrCl < 35
Propafenone	**IV** 1.5–2 mg/kg over 10–20 min **Oral** IR: 150–300 mg q 8 h ER: 225–425 mg q 12 h (Oral LD 450 mg (wt < 70 kg)–600 mg (wt > 70 kg), MD 450–900 mg/d divided into q 8 h (IR), or 12 h (ER))	Sinus or AV node dysfunction or Infranodal conduction disease HF CAD Atrial flutter Brugada syndrome Liver disease Asthma may cause dysgeusia	Metabolized by CYP2D6 (inhibitors include quinidine, fluoxetine, tricyclics; also genetically absent in 7–10% of population)—poor metabolizers have ⇧beta blockade Inhibits P-glycoprotein: ⇧digoxin concentration Inhibits CYP2C9: ⇧warfarin concentration (⇧INR 25%) Decrease dose in hepatic failure
Vaughan Williams class III			
Amiodarone	**IV** LD 150 mg over 10 min; followed by 1 mg/min for 6 h; then 0.5 mg/min for 18 h or change to oral dosing; after 24 h, consider decreasing dose to 0.25 mg/min **Oral** 400–600 mg daily in divided doses for 2–4 wk; maintenance typically 100–200 mg QD	Sinus or AV node dysfunction Infranodal conduction disease Lung disease Prolonged QT interval	Inhibits most CYPs to cause drug interaction: ⇧concentrations of warfarin (⇧INR between 0–200%), statins, many other drugs Inhibits P-glycoprotein: ⇧digoxin concentration

Drug	Usual doses	Side effects sects	Additional information
Dronedarone	**Oral** 400 mg BID	Bradycardia HF Liver disease Thyriod disease pulmonary fibrosis Prolonged QT interval	Metabolized by CYP3A: caution with inhibitors (e.g., verapamil, diltiazem, ketoconazole, macrolide antibiotics, protease inhibitors, grapefruit juice) and inducers (e.g., phenytoin, phenobarbital, rifampin) Inhibits CYP3A, CYP2D6, P-glycoprotein: ⇧concentrations of some statins, digoxin, beta blockers, sirolimus, tacrolimus Avoid in long-standing persistent or permanent AF and HF
Dofetilide	**Oral** 125–500 mcg BID if CrCl >60, 250 mcg if CrCl 40–60, 125 mcg if CrCl 20–40 Decrease MD if QTc increased by >15% of >500 ms 2–3 h after dose or consider discontinuing it	Prolonged QT interval and torsades de pointes Renal disease Hypokalemia hypomagnesaemia AV block, bradycardia, sick sinus syndrome	Adjust dose for renal function, body size, and age (avoid if CrCl < 20) Drug interactions via CYP3A4: CI to use with verapamil, cimetidine, ketoconazole, trimethoprim, prochlorperazine, HCTZ, and megestrol Discontinue amiodarone at least 3 m before initiation Avoid other QT interval prolonging drugs
Ibutilide	**IV** 1 mg over 10 min; may repeat 1 mg once if necessary (if weight <60 kg, use 0.01 mg/kg)	Prolonged QT interval and torsade de pointes hypotension CAD HF	Mointor K and mg level
Sotalol	**Oral** 40–160 mg q12 h **IV** 75–150 mg QD or BID over 5 h (only if patient cannot take oral)	Prolonged QT interval Sinus or AV nodal dysfunction HF	Renal excretion: CI if Cr Cl <40 decrease dose if CrCl 40–60 Risk of torsade de pointes (do not initiate sotalol therapy if the baseline QTc is longer than 450 ms. If the QT interval prolongs to 500 ms or greater, the dose must be reduced, the duration of the infusion prolonged or the drug discontinued) Avoid other QT interval prolonging drugs correct hypokalemia/hypomagnesemia

ACC AF [74]; JACC [53]. AF, atrial fibrillation; AV, atrioventricular; BID, twice daily; CAD, coronary artery disease; CI, contraindicated; CrCl, creatinine clearance; ER, extended release; h, hour; HCTZ, hydrochlorothiazide; HF, heart failure; IL, immediate release; IV, intravenous; LD, loading dose; INR, international normalized ratio; MD, maintenance dose; min, minute; max, maximum; SLE, systemic lupus erythematosus; Q, every; QD, once daily; wt, weight. http://www.pdr.net/

Table 2. Medications commonly used for atrial fibrillation Rythm Control with its dosage and major pharmacokinetic and drug interactions.

Oral anticoagulation at discharge has been associated with a reduced long-term mortality in patients with POAF [83] but without evidence from controlled trials [75]. POAF that persists for longer than 48 h should be anticoagulated with warfarin or nonvitamin K antagonist oral anticoagulants (NOACs). The NOACs are available for the treatment of nonvalvular AF. NOACs have been found to be as efficacious or even superior to warfarin in the prevention of stroke in nonvalvular AF patients with high risk of thromboembolism, with similar to lower rates of major bleeding, and also lower rates of intracranial hemorrhage [84].

3.1.6. Prevention of POAF

Beta-blockers are effective in reducing POAF and SVTs. Propranolol uses reduced POAF incidence from 31.7% in the control group to 16.3% in the treatment group [85]. In the majority of beta-blocker studies, it is administered postoperatively [86]. Amiodarone reduced the incidence of POAF and hospital stay compared to beta-blocker therapy in several meta-analyses [86–89]. Prophylactic administration of sotalol may be considered for patients at risk of developing AF after cardiac surgery [76, 90, 91]. Also, administration of colchicine postoperatively may reduce POAF [75, 92]. Statin use preoperatively did not prevent POAF in a prospective controlled trial [93], despite that initial reports from meta-analyses were encouraging [94–96].

Other therapies for the prevention of POAF have been studied in small trials, but have not demonstrated clear beneficial effects [76]. These include angiotensin converting enzyme inhibitors (ACEIs) [97], magnesium [85, 98, 99], n-3 polyunsaturated fatty acids [100–108], corticosteroids [109–111], and posterior pericardiectomy [112]. Conflicting results have also been reported for acetylcysteine [113], and sodium nitroprusside [114].

Nonpharmacologic therapy with atrial pacing has been tested in various studies [7]. One meta-analysis showed a significant reduction in POAF with atrial pacing (OR 0.57, 95% CI 0.38–0.84) [67], and most [115–117] but not all [118, 119] published studies showed benefit with this therapy. Besides, there are conflicting findings as to the relative value of the different types of atrial pacing [115, 116].

3.2. Postoperative atrial flutter (POAFL)

Unlike POAF, POAFL after CABG is not well studied. In a single-center study with 80 consecutive patients who underwent CABG with no previous history of AFL, 16 patients (20%) had documented POAFL. Ten of these patients showed temporary AFLs that were curable without radiofrequency catheter ablation (RFCA), and 37.5% of the patients with POAFL (i.e., 7.5% of the patients after CABG) showed sustained or repeated AFL with subjective symptoms [120]. In another study that looked at ATs late after open heart surgery, it was found that cavotricuspid isthmus (CTI)-dependent AFL was the most common. Atypical AFL becomes progressively more widespread with more extensive atriotomy [121]. AFL and ATs that developed late after cardiac surgery are believed to be due to scars created by incisions applied to the right and/or left atrium either for establishing extracorporeal circulation or access to intracardiac structures (coronary sinus, interatrial or interventricular septum, atrioventricular valves, etc.) [122]. The scars created by these incisions play a significant role in the development of ATs, months or years after surgery [123, 124].

AFL in the early postoperative period is managed as POAF with rate control or rhythm control and anticoagulation based on arrhythmia duration and patient risk factors. On long-term catheter ablation of AFL is an effective, safe, and potentially curative procedure.

3.3. Supraventricular tachycardia (SVT)

3.3.1. Epidemiology

Sinus tachycardia (ST) represents an appropriate autonomic response to a physiological stress. The upper limit of normal rate for sinus tachycardia is calculated from the formula

(220 bpm minus age) [125]. Inappropriate ST may be seen in some patients, especially with young age, but it is rare and should be considered a diagnosis of exclusion [125]. The term 'SVT' refers to paroxysmal tachyarrhythmias that require atrial or AV nodal tissue, or both, for their initiation and maintenance [126]. It is typical of a sudden or paroxysmal onset and includes AV nodal reentrant tachycardias (AVNRT), AV reentrant tachycardias (AVRT), and atrial tachycardias. The overall incidence of perioperative arrhythmias in noncardiac surgery varies from 16 to 62% with intermittent ECG monitoring and up to 89% with continuous Holter monitoring [127]. It is more likely to be supraventricular than ventricular in origin [127]. In small study, the incidence of persistent SVT in noncardiac surgery patients was 2% during surgery and 6% in the postoperative period [128].

3.3.2. Diagnosis

12-lead ECG and rhythm strips during tachycardia are diagnostic and may give an impression about the most likely diagnosis. Although ST is usually easy to diagnose on 12-lead ECG, the presence of first-degree AV block, which is not uncommon after cardiac surgery, may give ECG appearance that mimics SVT due to P wave merge with T wave (P wave hidden within T wave). ECG features of ATs including SVTs are shown in **Table 3**.

3.3.3. Clinical course

ATs occur most frequently 2–3 days postsurgery and are likely related to sympathetic stimulation associated with an inflammatory response [129]. Patients with known SVT may have an exacerbation of their tachycardia in the perioperative period. However, SVT may be diagnosed for the first time in the perioperative period [2, 7, 130, 131]. SVT is often associated with a high sympathetic tone, but other precipitants may contribute to its occurrence. The clinical symptoms, time of onset, and natural course of ATs are identical in patients with cardiac, thoracic, or other surgery.

3.3.4. Prognosis

The prognosis of perioperative SVTs is good, but it may be associated with increased hospital stay [128].

3.3.5. Management

The SVT management, in general, depends on the hemodynamic status of the patient. If the patient with SVT is hemodynamically unstable, synchronized cardioversion is recommended for acute termination of the tachycardia when vagal maneuvers or adenosine is ineffective or not feasible [132]. Before initiating specific drug therapy for acute SVT in hemodynamically stable patients, it is important to assess and correct possible precipitating factors such as respiratory failure or electrolyte imbalance. SVT may respond to vagal maneuver if the patient can do it. Adenosine might be used if there is no contraindication. SVT also responds to rate control drugs such as beta-blockers (e.g., esmolol, metoprolol, bisoprolol) or nondihydropyridine calcium channel antagonists (e.g., diltiazem, verapamil). Intravenous (IV) digoxin, IV amiodarone, adenosine, IV or oral beta-blockers, diltiazem, and verapamil are potentially harmful in acute treatment in patients with pre-excited AF (AF in patients with Wolff-Parkinson-White (WPW) syndrome) [133]. Of note, atrial tachycardia unifocal or multifocal usually respond to rate control drugs but are not amenable to direct current cardioversion. Cardiac electrophysiology study with catheter ablation is an effective long-term management for recurrent SVT.

4. Postoperative ventricular tachyarrhythmias (POVTAs)

The postoperative ventricular tachyarrhythmias (POVTAs) range from isolated PVC to VT or ventricular fibrillation (VF).

4.1. Premature ventricular complexes (PVCs)

4.1.1. Epidemiology

Isolated PVCs including nonsustained ventricular tachycardia (NSVT) are seen in about 50% of patients during and after cardiac surgery [134]. PVCs can be related to electrolyte or other metabolic imbalances [7].

4.1.2. Diagnosis

PVCs may be seen on continuous telemetric monitoring and 12-lead ECG, however, careful evaluation of the ECG tracing is needed to be distinguished from atrial ectopy with aberrant ventricular conduction [7].

4.1.3. Clinical course

Patients with postoperative PVCs may be asymptomatic or may have palpitations with a skipped beat, or dizziness. It is rarely associated with hemodynamic instability.

4.1.4. Prognosis

Patients with isolated and noncomplicated PVCs postoperatively do not exhibit increased risk of malignant VAs [135, 136]. On the contrary, frequent PVCs (>30 per hour) may reduce ventricular function and therefore have an adverse impact on the short-term outcome. There was no significant difference in mortality in patients with versus patients without frequent postoperative PVCs and NSVT (8 versus 5%), at an average follow-up of 3 years, in a study including 185 postoperative patients [137]. However, in another study of 126 patients with postoperative PVCs, it was shown that patients with left ventricular ejection fraction (LVEF) of <40% had a 75% mortality rate and 33% incidence of sudden death at an average follow-up of 15 months, whereas none of the patients with preserved left ventricular function had sudden death [135]. Thus, PVCs are not related to mortality with good LV function, and long-term outcome after cardiac surgery seems to be closely related to the left ventricular function.

4.1.5. Management

Correction of any reversible cause of ventricular arrhythmias should be performed. Hemo dynamically stable and asymptomatic PVCs do not usually need treatment with antiarrhythmic therapy on short or long-term. Lidocaine has been used with a successful result in reducing hemodynamically significant or symptomatic PVCs, but without improving mortality. Empirical use of class I antiarrhythmic drugs for suppression of frequent and/or complex PVCs had no beneficial effects on mortality rate and may be harmful as shown in several studies in another setting [138, 139]. Additionally, overdrive pacing, using either atrial or atrioventricular sequential pacing, has been used without significant results [138, 139]. Patients with asymptomatic NSVT after cardiac surgery and preserved LVEF generally have a favorable long-term prognosis and do not require invasive workup with an electrophysiology study. The use of implantable cardioverter defibrillators (ICDs) has shown no benefits in improving prognosis in this population [140].

4.2. Ventricular tachyarrhythmias

4.2.1. Epidemiology

Sustained VT and VF rarely occur after cardiac surgery with an incidence of 0.4–1.7% in most of the studies [138, 141], but an incidence of 3.1% has been reported [142]. Furthermore, it is life threatening and affects outcome [134, 143].

4.2.2. Pathophysiology and risk factors

Pathophysiology of POAs, in general, was disused in item 2. Coronary artery disease (CAD) leads to a broad spectrum of changes and may trigger arrhythmia mechanisms via enhanced automaticity, triggered activity, and reentry. While myocardial infarction (MI) related scar constitutes the clinical model of reentry [144], focal activation due to abnormal automaticity is the primary mechanism involved in the VT during acute ischemia [145]. Early and delayed after depolarization result from focal discharge by calcium overload and triggered activity is another likely mechanism of VT initiation in ischemia, but this needs to be proven experimentally thus far [146, 147]. Acute ischemia activates the adenosine triphosphate-sensitive potassium (K-ATP) channels, causing an increase in extracellular potassium along with acidosis and hypoxia in the cardiac muscle. As a result of the minor increases in extracellular potassium depolarize the myocardiocyte's resting membrane potential, which can increase tissue excitability in early phases of ischemia [145]. The mechanism underlying the VT associated with healed or healing MI is reentry in more than 95% of cases [144].

Complex ventricular arrhythmias (VAs) are associated with multiple risk factors [7]. Based on clinical studies, the conditions associated with VAs after cardiac surgery may include: increased age, female gender, presence of unstable angina, congestive cardiac failure, hemodynamic instability, preoperative use of inotropes, preoperative use of IABP, emergency surgery, electrolyte disturbances, hypoxia, hypovolemia, myocardial ischemia/infarction, acute graft closure, reperfusion after cessation of CPB, and inotropes antiarrhythmic drugs use, on-pump surgery, and PVD [134, 135, 141, 143, 148].

	Heart rate (bpm)	Regularity	Onset	Atrial activity	Response to adenosine	Rhythm strip
AF	A: 350-500 V: 100- 220	Irregular	Sudden	No discrete P-waves	Transient slowing of ventricular rate	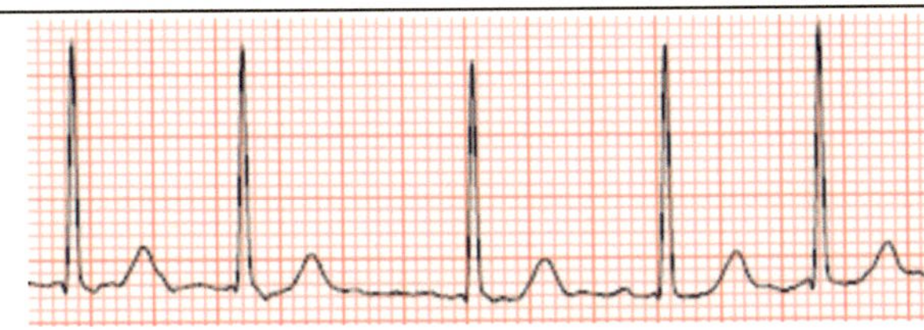
AFL	A: 250-350 V: 150 (slower or faster depends on AV conduction)	Regular (irregular with variable AV conduction)	Sudden	Flutter waves "saw-tooth" pattern)	Transient slowing of ventricular rate	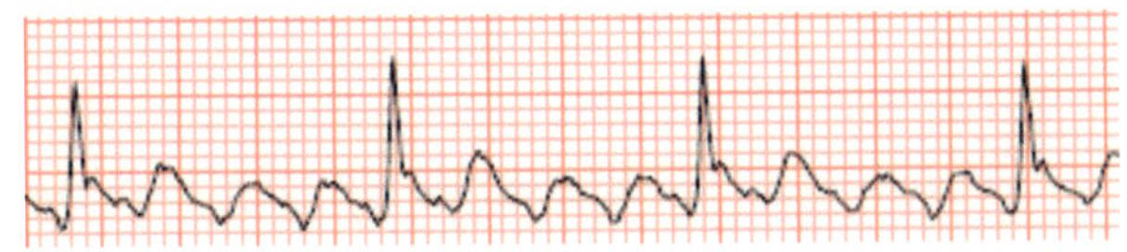
ST	220-age	Regular	Gradual	Normal P-waves	Transient slowing	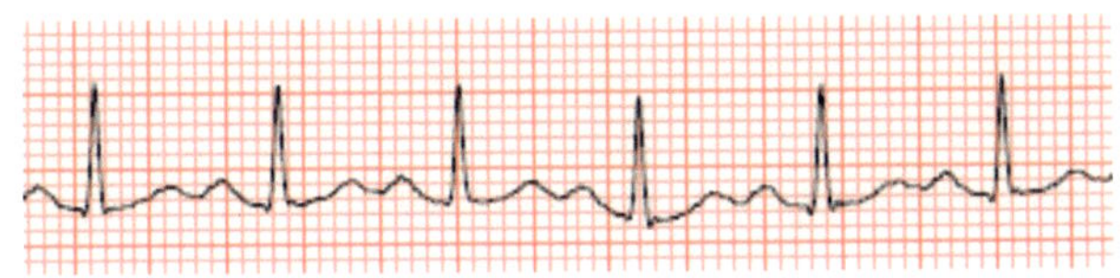
AT	150-250	Regular	Sudden	Abnormal P-waves morphology	-Transient slowing of ventricular rate -May terminate tachycardia in 70% of the cases	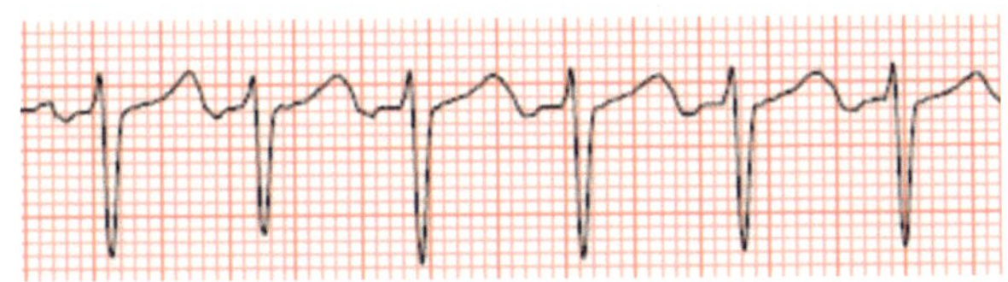
AVNRT	150-250	Regular	Sudden	No obvious P-waves as P- wave is in or just after QRS (Pseudo r′ in V1 or S wave in inferior leads)	Termination of tachycardia	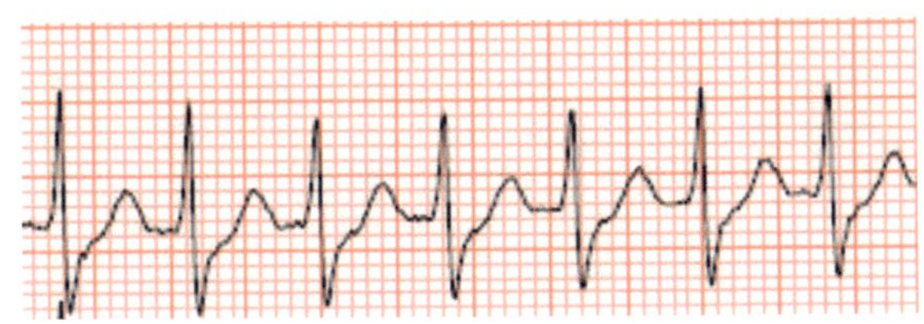

	Heart rate (bpm)	Regularity	Onset	Atrial activity	Response to adenosine	Rhythm strip
AVRT (WPW)	150-250	Regular	Sudden	**ORT:** P-waves may be buried in QRS complex, or retrograde P wave may be seen at the end of the QRS complex or in the early part of the ST segment	Termination of tachycardia	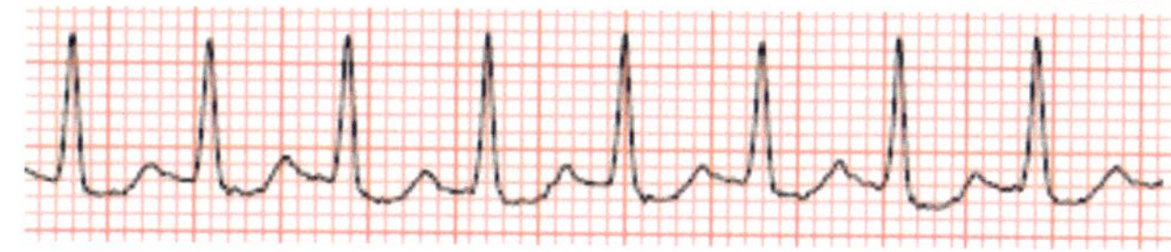
				ART: P wave normal with short PR and delta wave (wide QRS complexes due to abnormal ventricular depolarization via accessory pathway)	Termination of tachycardia	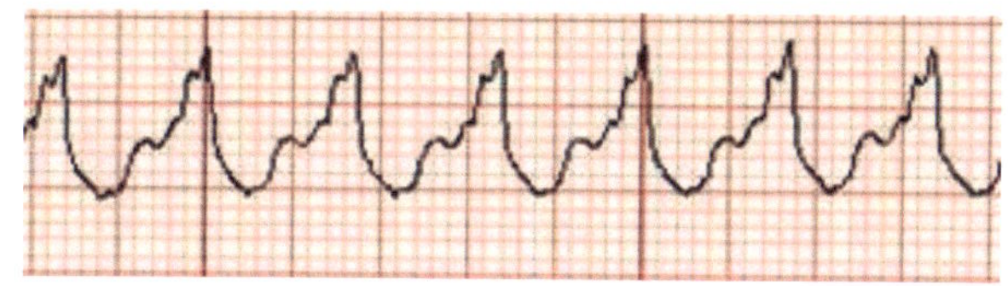
				AF: no P-wave, irregular rhythm, and wide QRS complex	Should not be used	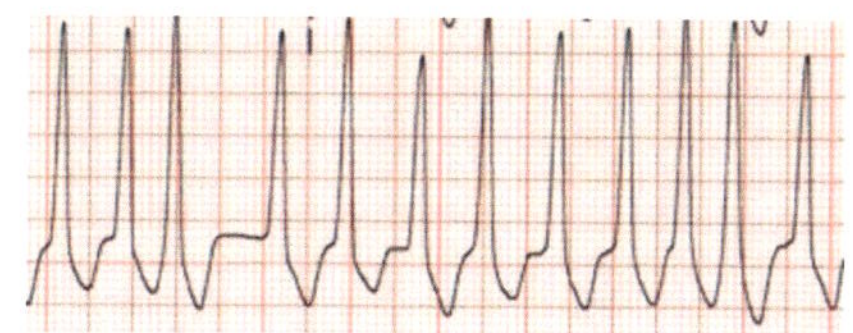

Table 3. Differential diagnosis of atrial tachyarrhythmias.

4.2.3. Diagnosis

In addition to a clinical history and a physical exam, the general evaluation of a patient with CAD and suspected or documented VAs includes performing a 12-lead ECG and an echocardiogram. Telemetry monitoring with careful evaluation of VAs initiation and termination is very helpful. Based on ECG criteria, wide complex tachycardias (WCT) may be either ventricular or SVT with aberrancy. However, in patients with structural heart disease like prior infarction, the diagnosis is mostly VT. If feasible, a 12-lead ECG and atrial electrograms through temporary epicardial wires placed at the time of cardiac surgery should be obtained. The presence of AV dissociation strongly suggests VT [138]. Although the ECG diagnosis of a WCT is challenging, it is important to remember that VT is the cause in at least 80% of cases [149].

4.2.4. Clinical course

Clinical presentation of patients post cardiac surgery with VTs is variable. The hemodynamic state of these patients depends mainly on the rate of the tachyarrhythmia and the left ventricular function. Therefore, some patients may be asymptomatic. Other patients with VT may complain of palpitations, dyspnea, or chest discomfort as their main symptoms. VTs may present with syncope and sudden cardiac death as a result of hemodynamic compromise. Incessant VT, even if it is hemodynamically stable, can lead to hemodynamic deterioration and heart failure [150, 151].

4.2.5. Prognosis

The prognosis is correlated with the type of arrhythmia and the type and degree of structural heart disease [7]. As mentioned earlier, PVCs and NSVT generally have no impact on the outcome. However, patients with sustained VAs have poorer short- and long-term prognosis.

POVAs predicts higher in-hospital mortality (21.7–31.5%) compared with (1.4–2.9%) in control [134, 143, 148]. In one study, POVAs was associated with increased long-term mortality over a mean follow-up of 3.5 years. Patients with POVAs had a high risk of death in the POVAs group during the first 6 postsurgical months (6-month survival of POVAs 59.8 versus 93.8% for POVAs free group). This difference in survival persisted over time [148].

4.2.6. Management of POVAs

Asymptomatic PVCs and hemodynamically stable short runs of NSVT do not need specific intervention, and the correction of any reversible cause of VAs is generally sufficient. Postoperative sustained VAs treatment follows the ICD indications used in other clinical settings [150, 152]. However, the postoperative patients require close attention to the identification and treatment of reversible causes of arrhythmia like electrolyte or other metabolic disturbances, myocardial ischemia, or mechanical complications of surgery [7]. Sustained VAs should be promptly cardioverted either by drugs infusion or electrically based on hemodynamic stability. Hemodynamically stable sustained VTs may be initially treated with antiarrhythmic drugs infusion.

4.2.6.1. Pharmacological treatment

It includes antiarrhythmic medication use and standard medical therapy. The most commonly used antiarrhythmic agents include:

- Amiodarone: IV amiodarone is frequently used as a first-line treatment for VAs as it is better tolerated in patients with low ejection fraction than the other antiarrhythmic drugs. The recommended starting dose of Cordarone I.V. is 1000 mg over the first 24 h of therapy. It is usually delivered by bolus infusion of 150 mg over 10–15 min, followed by 1 mg/min for 6 h, then 0.5 mg/min infusion for 18 h. The alternative dose would be 300 mg over 1 h then infusion at 50 mg/h. Additional 150 mg blouses may be given but frequent boluses during the first 24 h should be limited due to the risk of hepatic toxicity [153].

- Lidocaine: it is generally a good choice if ischemia is suspected. Lidocaine is administered as a bolus of 0.75–1.5 mg/kg, followed by an IV infusion of 1–4 mg/min (the maximal dose is 3 mg/kg/h). In elderly patient and patients with congestive heart failure or hepatic dysfunction, the lidocaine dose should be reduced [153].

- Procainamide: it is often a second line drug, and it is given as loading dose of 15–18 mg/kg administered as a slow infusion over 25–30 min or 100 mg/dose. The infusion rate should not exceed 50 mg/min. The loading dose may be repeated every 5 min as needed to a total dose of 1 g. However, it should be stopped if hypotension occurs, or QRS complex widens by 50% of its original width. This is followed by a maintenance dose of 1–4 mg/min by continuous infusion. The procainamide maintenance infusion should be reduced by 1/3 in patients with moderate renal or cardiac impairment and by 2/3 in patients with severe renal or cardiac impairment [153].

Standard medical therapy includes beta-blockers, and ACEIs drugs have been demonstrated to improve long-term survival particularly in patients with left ventricular dysfunction.

4.2.6.2. Nonpharmacological management

- Overdrive pacing: in patients with slower VTs who have ventricular epicardial wires, overdrive pacing may be performed. Electrical cardioversion/defibrillation should be easily available because of the possibility of acceleration of the VT or degeneration to VF [154].

- Electrical cardioversion/defibrillation: in patients with cardiac arrest, basic life support (BLS) and advanced cardiovascular life support (ACLS) should be followed. Electrical defibrillation should be performed for VF, pulseless VT, and hemodynamically unstable VT. Electrical cardioversion may be used for stable sustained VT as the first choice or for those who do not respond to antiarrhythmic medications. The recommended energy with current biphasic defibrillators ranges from 150 to 200 Joules. Sedation with short-acting agents should precede cardioversion in awake patients [154].

- Emergency mechanical support: in postoperative patients who are not responding to standard resuscitation maneuvers, initiation of emergency CPB in the intensive care unit may be considered. In one study, CPB use in a postoperative cardiac arrest was associated with a 56% long-term survival rate with a 22% incidence of soft tissue infections and no mediastinitis [154].

- Implantable cardioverter-defibrillator (ICD) therapy:

In the absence of a reversible cause of sustained VT or cardiac arrest after CABG, long-term management may include electrophysiology study and eventually an ICD implantation. Patients with NSVT, prior MI, and left ventricular dysfunction (LVEF <40%) may be considered for electrophysiology testing and implantation of an ICD if a sustained ventricular arrhythmia is induced [152, 155]. Multicenter automatic defibrillator implantation trial (MADIT) study [152] excluded subjects within 2 months after CABG and 3 months after percutaneous transluminal coronary angioplasty (PTCA), and MADIT-II study [156] excluded subjects within 3 months after revascularization. Conversely, early revascularization was permitted in MUSTT (Multicenter Unsustained Tachycardia Trial) study [155], which enrolled subjects at least 4 days after revascularization, and sudden cardiac death in heart failure trial (SCD-HeFT) study [157] made no specific exclusion on the timing of revascularization. However, in SCD-HeFT, the median time from CABG to enrollment was 3.1 years, and from PCI to enrollment was 2.3 years. Therefore, ICD implantation within 90 days of coronary revascularization for patients who otherwise meet ICD implant criteria for primary prevention of sudden cardiac death (SCD) is not addressed in the published device-based therapy guidelines. Revascularization has significant time-dependent benefits. In fact, MADIT-II study showed that the efficacy of ICD therapy in patients with ischemic left ventricular dysfunction is time dependent, with a significant life-saving benefit in patients receiving device implantation more than 6 months after coronary revascularization (CR). The lack of ICD benefit early after CR may be related to a relatively small risk of SCD during this period [158]. Although, sudden cardiac arrest (SCA) has a higher incidence in patients with reduced LVEF in the months after acute MI and/or following revascularization [159, 160]. The two randomized controlled trials, defibrillator in acute myocardial infarction (DINAMIT) and immediate risk stratification improves survival (IRIS), showed that early ICD implantation does not reduce mortality [161, 162]. In both of those trials, there was a reduction in arrhythmic death, which was counteracted by a concomitant increase in death due to other causes [163]. Similarly, the coronary artery bypass graft (CABG)-patch trial [164] examined ICD implantation at the time of elective CABG surgery showed a small decrease in arrhythmic death, but no benefit for overall mortality in patients with preoperative LVEF ≤35%. However, one should keep in mind that the epicardial ICDs tested in this trial differed significantly from the current transvenous endocardial ICD systems. A retrospective study evaluating ICD implantation within 3 months of cardiac surgery suggested the benefit of ICD implantation for secondary prevention. In this study, 164 patients were with ICD implantation within 3 months of cardiac surgery; 93 of these patients had an ICD for sustained pre or postoperative VT or VF requiring resuscitation. During the mean follow-up of 49 months; the primary endpoint was total mortality (TM) and/or appropriate ICD therapy (ICD-T), and secondary endpoints are the TM and ICD-T, and individual end points of TM and ICD-T were observed in 52 (56%), 35 (38%), and 28 (30%) patients, respectively, with 55% of TM, and 23% of ICD-T occurring within 2 years of implant [165].

Overall, ICD for *primary prevention* of SCD *can be useful* in patients who are within 90 days of revascularization and who are not within 40 days of an acute MI if:

- they are previously qualified for primary prevention of SCD or

- revascularization is unlikely to result in an improvement in LVEF to level >35% [166].

ICD for *secondary prevention* (i.e., in patients resuscitated from cardiac arrest due to VT/VF) *is recommended* for patients within 90 days of revascularization who have:

- previously satisfied criteria for ICD implantation if they have abnormal left ventricular function or

- SCD is unlikely related to myocardial ischemia/injury and have normal left ventricular function [166].

ICD implantation *can be useful* in patients who are within 90 days of revascularization if SCD was not related to acute myocardial ischemia/injury and who were subsequently found to have coronary artery disease that is revascularized with normal left ventricular function, or SCD was not related to acute myocardial ischemia/injury and who were subsequently found to have coronary artery disease that is revascularized with normal left ventricular function [166]. ICD is *not recommended* in patients within 90 days of revascularization who were resuscitated from cardiac arrest due to VT that was related to acute MI/injury, with normal left ventricular function, and who undergo complete coronary revascularization [166]. ICD with appropriately selected pacing capabilities *is recommended* in patients within 90 days of revascularization who require nonelective permanent pacing, who would also meet primary prevention criteria for implantation of an ICD, and in whom recovery of left ventricular function is uncertain or not expected [166].

An alternative approach for primary prevention of SCD in patients with ischemic cardiomyopathy and low LVEF undergoing revascularization would be the use the wearable cardioverter-defibrillator vest during the 3 months waiting period after revascularization until LVEF is reassessed and design made about permanent ICD implantation [163].

- Ventricular tachycardia ablation:

There are no studies of VT ablation in POVAs situation. In patients with extensive structural abnormalities, especially those with prior MI, multiple morphologies of VT might develop. Therefore, VT ablation does not eliminate the need for ICD and/or antiarrhythmic therapy. VT episodes might occur in up 0–60% of patients who have received an ICD for secondary prevention and in 2.5–12% of patients with ICD implanted for primary prevention [167]. Because antiarrhythmic drugs do not eliminate the risk of VAs, VT catheter ablation may be needed to reduce the frequency of VT episodes, especially patients with incessant VT or frequent ICD therapy [149]. Ablation is usually indicated in cases of recurrent, monomorphic VT arising from a specific substrate that can be targeted by mapping techniques.

5. Postoperative bradyarrhythmias (POBAs)

5.1. Epidemiology

Bradyarrhythmias (BAs) are common after cardiac surgery, but it mostly consists of transient episodes of low ventricular heart rate. The conduction defects post cardiac surgery include sinus node dysfunction, partial and complete bundle branch blocks, and various degrees of atrioventricular (AV) block. The right bundle branch block (RBBB) was the most frequently noted abnormality [168]. Bradyarrhythmias may decrease cardiac output in patients with relatively fixed stroke volumes. The risk of developing conduction disturbances after CABG or valvular surgery leading to permanent pacemaker (PPM) implantation is about 0.4–1.1% of patients after isolated CABG and 3–6% after heart valve operations [169–171]. It seems that in the current surgical era that the incidence of postoperative PPM implantation has decreased due to improvements in surgical techniques, technological innovations and enhanced understanding of the mechanisms of injury [172]. However, some studies have shown an increased incidence of PPM implantation after cardiac surgery after the year 2000 [173].

5.2. Pathophysiology and risk factors

Conduction disorders after cardiac surgery are explained by one of the following two mechanisms: (1) direct trauma to the conduction system in operative procedures in proximity to the sinoatrial or AV nodes or the His bundle; or (2) ischemic injury to the conduction system due to extensive coronary artery disease might compromise myocardial protection during intraoperative cardioplegic arrest [174].

The risk factors for POBAs may be classified as preoperative, operative, and postoperative factors. Preoperative risk factors include age >75 years, the use of rate lowering cardiac medications (e.g., beta-blockers, calcium channel blockers, digoxin, and antiarrhythmic drugs), the presence of conduction system disease preoperatively, right bundle branch block (RBBB) or left bundle branch block (LBBB), first-degree AV block or left anterior fascicular block (LAFB) [169–171, 175–178].

Operative risk factors include myocardial ischemia, inadequate cardiac protection during surgery, and direct surgical injury to conduction system, prolonged CPB time and cross-clamp time, and reoperation [171, 172, 174, 179, 180].

Postoperative risk factors include postoperative conduction disturbances and high-grade AV block [174, 175, 181].

5.3. Clinical course and management

Temporary electrical pacing may be required in symptomatic bradycardias. It is common practice nowadays to place temporary epicardial atrial and ventricular pacing wires placed at the time of surgery to facilitate temporary pacing when needed. In some cases, as mentioned above, the conduction defect does not revert, and permanent pacing may be necessary. Chronotropic medications, such as theophylline or aminophylline, have been used for sinus bradycardia after transplantation to improve SSS [182] or high-grade AVB [183] and may decrease the need for permanent pacing but its long-term effect is not encouraging.

The challenge with POBAs is often to determine when to implant the PPM as the sinus node function or AV conduction may recover in some patients. Recovery of conduction system is common with long-term follow-up. Only 30–40% of patients with a permanent pacemaker due to sinus node disease remain pacemaker dependent. However, the rate of recovery is less in patients with postoperative AVB, as 65–100% of patients with complete heart block, remain pacemaker dependent. Currently, the usual practice is to implant a PPM if postoperative symptomatic complete AVB or severe sinus node dysfunction persists longer than 5–7 days [184]. PPM implantation may be considered earlier if the underlying intrinsic rhythm is absent or temporary pacing leads fail.

6. Conclusion

Arrhythmias are common after CABG. Although tachyarrhythmias are frequent, they are usually transient and have a benign course. POAF represents the most frequently observed ATs. VAs are less common but have an adverse impact on the short and long-term outcome. POTAs management includes optimization of the patient's condition, controlling patient's risk factors, and careful attention to hemodynamic changes during surgery with using appropriate anesthesia. Postoperatively, it is important to correct reversible arrhythmia predisposing factors, followed by specific therapy based on the arrhythmia type and its hemodynamic effect.

On the other hand, bradyarrhythmias are also frequently observed after cardiac surgery. However, most of the conduction disturbances are transient and recovered spontaneously. PPM implantation may be required in patients with persistent symptomatic bradycardia due to sick sinus syndrome or second degree type 2, third degree, or high-grade AV block.

Author details

Bandar Al-Ghamdi[1,2]*

*Address all correspondence to: balghamdi@kfshrc.edu.sa

1 Heart Centre, King Faisal Specialist Hospital and Research Centre, Riyadh, Saudi Arabia

2 College of Medicine, Alfaisal University, Riyadh, Saudi Arabia

References

[1] Herzog L, Lynch C. Arrhythmias accompanying cardiac surgery. In: Lynch C, editor. Clinical Cardiac Electrophysiology. 3rd ed. Philadelphia, PA, USA: JB Lippincott; 1994. pp. 231-258.

[2] Creswell LL, Schuessler RB, Rosenbloom M, Cox JL. Hazards of postoperative atrial arrhythmias. The Annals of Thoracic Surgery. 1993;**56**:539-549. DOI: https://doi.org/10.1016/0003-4975(93)90894-N

[3] Mathew JP, Fontes ML, Tudor IC, Ramsay J, Duke P, Mazer CD, Barash PG, Hsu PH, Mangano DT, Investigators of the Ischemia Research and Education Foundation, Multicenter Study of Perioperative Ischemia Research Group. A multicenter risk index for atrial fibrillation after cardiac surgery. JAMA. 2004;**291**:1720-1729. DOI: 10.1001/jama.291.14.1720

[4] Steinbach K, Merl O, Frohner K, Hief C, Nurnberg M, Kalten-brunner W, Podczeck A, Wessely E. Hemodynamics during ventricular tachyarrhythmias. American Heart Journal. 1994;**127**:1102-1106. DOI: http://dx.doi.org/10.1016/0002-8703(94)90095-7

[5] Fenelon G, Wigjns W, Andries E, Brugada P. Tachycardiomyopathy: Mechanisms and clinical implications. PACE. 1996;**19**:95-106. DOI: 10.1111/j.1540-8159.1996.tb04796.x

[6] Baig MW, Perrins EJ. The hemodynamics of cardiac pacing. Progress in Cardiovascular Diseases. 1991;**33**:283-298. DOI: https://doi.org/10.1016/0033-0620(91)90021-D

[7] Peretto G, Durante A, Limite LR, Cianflone D. Postoperative arrhythmias after cardiac surgery: Incidence, risk factors, and therapeutic management. Cardiology Research and Practice. 2014;**2014**:615987. DOI: 10.1155/2014/615987

[8] Diodato M, Chedrawy EG. Coronary artery bypass graft surgery: The past, present, and future of myocardial revascularisation. Surgery Research and Practice. 2014;**2014**:726158. DOI: 10.1155/2014/726158

[9] Møller CH, Penninga L, Wetterslev J, Steinbruchel DA, Gluud C. Off-pump versus on-pump coronary artery bypass grafting for ischaemic heart disease. Cochrane Database of Systematic Reviews. 2012 March 14;**3**:CD007224. DOI: 10.1002/14651858.CD007224.pub2

[10] Mack M, Acuff T, Yong P, Jett GK, Carter D. Minimally invasive thoracoscopically assisted coronary artery bypass surgery. European Journal of Cardio-Thoracic Surgery. 1997;**12**:20-24. DOI: https://doi.org/10.1016/S1010-7940(97)00141-3

[11] Enríquez F, Jiménez A. Post-operative tachyarrhythmias in adult cardiac surgery: Prophylaxis. Cirugia Cardiovascular. 2010;**17**:259-274. DOI: Https://doi.org/10.1016/S1134-0096(10)70100-5 (in Spanish: Taquiarritmias postoperatorias en la cirugía cardíaca del adulto. Profilaxis)

[12] Zaman AG, Archbold RA, Helft G, Atrial Paul EA, Curzen NP, Mills PG. Atrial fibrillation after coronary artery bypass surgery: A model for preoperative risk stratification. Circulation. 2000;**101**:1403-1408. DOI: https://doi.org/10.1161/01.CIR.101.12.1403

[13] Leitch JW, Thomson D, Baird DK, Harris PJ. The importance of age as a predictor of atrial fibrillation and flutter after coronary artery bypass grafting. The Journal of Thoracic and Cardiovascular Surgery. 1990;**100**:338-342 PMID: 2391970

[14] Premaratne S, Premaratne ID, Fernando ND, Williams L, Hasaniya NW. Atrial fibrillation and flutter following coronary artery bypass graft surgery: A retrospective study and review. JRSM Cardiovascular Disease. 2016;**5**:2048004016634149. DOI: 10.1177/2048004016634149

[15] Mendes LA, Connelly GP, McKenney PA, Podrid PJ, Cupples LA, Shemin RJ, Ryan TJ, Davidoff R. Right coronary artery stenosis: An independent predictor of atrial fibrillation after coronary artery bypass surgery. Journal of the American College of Cardiology. 1995;**25**:198-202. DOI: https://doi.org/10.1016/0735-1097(94)00329-O

[16] Helgadottir S, Sigurdsson MI, Ingvarsdottir IL, Arnar DO, Gudbjartsson T. Atrial fibrillation following cardiac surgery: Risk analysis and long-term survival. Journal of Cardiothoracic Surgery. 2012;**7**:87. DOI: 10.1186/1749-8090-7-87

[17] Kolvekar S, D'Souza A, Akhtar P, Reek C, Garratt C, Spyt T. Role of atrial ischaemia in development of atrial fibrillation following coronary artery bypass surgery. European Journal of Cardio-Thoracic Surgery. 1997;**11**:70-75. DOI: 10.1016/S1010-7940(96)01095-0

[18] Wazni OM, Martin DO, Marrouche NF, Latif AA, Ziada K, Shaaraoui M, Almahameed S, Schweikert RA, Saliba WI, Gillinov AM, Tang WH, Mills RM, Francis GS, Young JB, Natale A. Plasma B-type natriuretic peptide levels predict postoperative atrial fibrillation in patients undergoing cardiac surgery. Circulation. 2004;**110**:124-127. DOI: https://doi.org/10.1161/01.CIR.0000134481.24511.BC

[19] Zacharias A, Schwann TA, Riordan CJ, Durham SJ, Shah AS, Habib RH. Obesity and risk of new-onset atrial fibrillation after cardiac surgery. Circulation. 2005;**112**:3247-3255 https://doi.org/10.1161/CIRCULATIONAHA.105.553743

[20] Maesen B, Nijs J, Maessen J, Allessie M, Schotten U. Post-operative atrial fibrillation: A maze of mechanisms. Europace. 2012;**14**:159-174. DOI: https://doi.org/10.1093/europace/eur208

[21] Warltier DC, Laffey JG, Boylan JF, Cheng DCH. The systemic inflammatory response to cardiac surgery: Implications for the anesthesiologist. Anesthesiology. 2002;**97**:215-252 PMID: 12131125

[22] Bulow NMH, Colpo E, Duarte MF, Correa EFM, Schlosser RS, Lauda A, Kade IJ, Rocha JBT. Inflammatory response in patients under coronary artery bypass grafting surgery and clinical implications: A review of the relevance of Dexmedetomidine use. ISRN Anesthesiology. 2014;**2014**:1-28 http://dx.doi.org/10.1155/2014/905238

[23] Prondzinsky R, Knüpfer A, Loppnow H, Redling F, Lehmann DW, Stabenow I, Witthaut R, Unverzagt S, Radke J, Zerkowski HR, Werdan K. Surgical trauma affects the proinflammatory status after cardiac surgery to a higher degree than cardiopulmonary bypass. The Journal of Thoracic and Cardiovascular Surgery. 2005;**129**:760-766. DOI: https://doi.org/10.1016/j.jtcvs.2004.07.052

[24] Angelini GD, Penny WJ, el-Ghamary F, West RR, Butchart EG. The incidence and significance of early pericardial effusion after open heart surgery. European Journal of Cardio-Thoracic Surgery. 1987;**1**:165-168. DOI: https://doi.org/10.1016/1010-7940(87)90034-0

[25] Stamou SC, Dangas G, Hill PC, Pfister AJ, Dullum MK, Boyce SW, Bafi AS, Garcia JM, Corso PJ. Atrial fibrillation after beating heart surgery. The American Journal of Cardiology. 2000;**86**:64-67. DOI: https://doi.org/10.1016/S0002-9149(00)00829-8

[26] Haïssaguerre M, Jaïs P, Shah DC, Takahashi A, Hocini M, Quiniou G, Garrigue S, Le Mouroux A, Le Métayer P, Clémenty J. Spontaneous initiation of atrial fibrillation by ectopic beats originating in the pulmonary veins. The New England Journal of Medicine. 1998;**339**:659-666. DOI: 10.1056/NEJM199809033391003

[27] Vinten-Johansen J. Involvement of neutrophils in the pathogenesis of lethal myocardial reperfusion injury. Cardiovascular Research. 2004;**61**:481-497. DOI: 10.1016/j.cardiores.2003.10.011

[28] Butler J, Parker D, Pillai R, Westaby S, Shale DJ, Rocker GM. Effects of cardiopulmonary bypass on systemic release of neutrophil elastase and tumour necrosis factor. The Journal of Thoracic and Cardiovascular Surgery. 1993;**105**:25-30 PMID:8419705

[29] Wakayama F, Fukuda I, Suzuki Y, Kondo N. Neutrophil elastase inhibitor, sivelestat, attenuates acute lung injury after cardiopulmonary bypass in the rabbit endotoxemia model. The Annals of Thoracic Surgery. 2007;**83**:153-160. DOI: 10.1016/j.athoracsur.2006.08.023

[30] Atlee JL. Perioperative cardiac dysrhythmias: Diagnosis and management. Anesthesiology. 1997;**86**:1397-1424

[31] Salazar C, Frishman W, Friedman S, Patel J, Lin YT, Oka Y, Frater RW, Becker RM. β-blockade therapy for supraventricular tachyarrhythmias after coronary surgery: A propranolol withdrawal syndrome? Angiology. 1979;**30**:816-819. DOI: 10.1177/000331977903001204

[32] Deliargyris EN, Raymond RJ, Guzzo JA, Dehmer GJ, Smith SC, Weiner MS, Roberts CS. Preoperative factors predisposing to early postoperative atrial fibrillation after isolated coronary artery bypass grafting. The American Journal of Cardiology. 2000;**85**:763-764. DOI: http://dx.doi.org/10.1016/S0002-9149(99)00857-7

[33] Rubin DA, Nieminski KE, Reed GE, Herman MV. Predictors, prevention, and long-term prognosis of atrial fibrillation after coronary artery bypass graft operations. The Journal of Thoracic and Cardiovascular Surgery. 1987;**94**:331-335 PMID: 3306163

[34] Tisdale JE, Patel R, Webb CR, Borzak S, Zarowitz BJ. Electrophysiologic and proarrhythmic effects of intravenous inotropic agents. Progress in Cardiovascular Diseases. 1995;**38**:167-180. DOI: http://dx.doi.org/10.1016/S0033-0620(05)80005-2

[35] Williams JB, Hernandez AF, Li S, Dokholyan RS, O'Brien SM, Smith PK, Ferguson TB, Peterson ED. Postoperative inotrope and vasopressor use following CABG: Outcome data from the CAPS-care study. Journal of Cardiac Surgery. 2011;**26**:572-578. DOI: 10.1111/j.1540-8191.2011.01301.x

[36] Haghjoo M. Pharmacological and nonpharmacological prevention of atrial fibrillation after coronary artery bypass surgery. The Journal of Tehran Heart Center. 2012;**7**:2-9 PMCID: PMC3466882

[37] Wahr JA, Parks R, Boisvert D, Comunale M, Fabian J, Ramsay J, Mangano DT. Preoperative serum potassium levels and perioperative outcomes in cardiac surgery patients. Multicenter study of perioperative ischemia research group. JAMA. 1999;**281**:2203-2210. DOI: 10.1001/jama.281.23.2203

[38] Luo X, Pan Z, Shan H, Xiao J, Sun X, Wang N, Lin H, Xiao L, Maguy A, Qi XY, Li Y, Gao X, Dong D, Zhang Y, Bai Y, Ai J, Sun L, Lu H, Luo XY, Wang Z, Lu Y, Yang B, Nattel S. MicroRNA-26 governs profibrillatory inward-rectifier potassium current changes in atrial fibrillation. The Journal of Clinical Investigation. 2013;**123**:1939-1951. DOI: 10.1172/JCI62185

[39] Pinski SL. Potassium replacement after cardiac surgery: It is not time to change practice, yet. Critical Care Medicine. 1999;**27**:2581-2582 PMID: 10579291

[40] England MR, Gordon G, Salem M, Chernow B. Magnesium administration and dysrhythmias after cardiac surgery: A placebo-controlled, double-blind, randomized trial. JAMA. 1992;**268**:2395-2402. DOI: 10.1001/jama.1992.03490170067027

[41] Aglio LS, Stanford GC, Maddi R, Boyd III JL, Nussbaum S, Chernow B. Hypomagnesemia is common following cardiac surgery. Journal of Cardiothoracic and Vascular Anesthesia. 1991;**5**:201-208. DOI: http://dx.doi.org/10.1016/1053-0770(91)90274-W

[42] Singh S, Johnson PI, Lee RE, Orfei E, Lonchyna VA, Sullivan HJ, Montoya A, Tran H, Wehrmacher WH, Wurster RD. Topography of cardiac ganglia in the adult human heart. The Journal of Thoracic and Cardiovascular Surgery. 1996;**112**:943-953. DOI: 10.1016/S0022-5223(96)70094-6

[43] Quan KJ, Lee JH, Geha AS, Biblo LA, Van Hare GF, Mackall JA, Carlson MD. Characterization of sinoatrial parasympathetic innervation in humans. Journal of Cardiovascular Electrophysiology. 1999;**10**:1060-1065. DOI: 10.1111/j.1540-8167.1999.tb00278.x

[44] Quan KJ, Lee JH, Van Hare GF, Biblo LA, Mackall JA, Carlson MD. Identification and characterization of atrioventricular parasympathetic innervation in humans. Journal of Cardiovascular Electrophysiology. 2002;**13**:735-739. DOI: 10.1046/j.1540-8167.2002.00735.x

[45] Carlson MD, Geha AS, Hsu J, Martin PJ, Levy MN, Jacobs G, Waldo AL. Selective stimulation of parasympathetic nerve fibers to the human sinoatrial node. Circulation. 1992;**85**:1311-1317. DOI: https://doi.org/10.1161/01.CIR.85.4.1311

[46] Cummings JE, Gill I, Akhrass R, Dery Biblo LA, Quan KJ. Preservation of the anterior fat pad paradoxically decreases the incidence of postoperative atrial fibrillation in humans. Journal of the American College of Cardiology. 2004;**17**(43):994-1000. DOI: 10.1016/j.jacc.2003.07.055

[47] CM W, Sander S, Coleman CI, Gallagher R, Takata H, Humphrey C, Henyan N, Gillespie EL, Kluger J. Impact of epicardial anterior fat pad retention on postcardiothoracic surgery atrial fibrillation incidence: The AFIST-III study. Journal of the American College of Cardiology. 2007;**49**:298-303. DOI: 10.1016/j.jacc.2006.10.033

[48] Mitchell LB. Incidence, timing and outcome of atrial tachyarrhythmias after cardiac surgery. In: Steinberg JS, editor. Atrial Fibrillation after Cardiac Surgery. Boston: Kluwer Academic Publishers; 2000. pp. 37-50.

[49] Maisel WH, Rawn JD, Stevenson WG. Atrial fibrillation after cardiac surgery. Annals of Internal Medicine. 2001;**135**:1061-1073. DOI: 10.7326/0003-4819-135-12-200112180-00010

[50] Blomstrom Lundqvist C. Post CABG atrial fibrillation: What are the incidence, predictors, treatment, and long-term outcome? In: Raviele A, editor. Cardiac Arrhythmias 2005. Venice, Italy: Springer; 2005. pp. 131-136.

[51] Pavri BB, O'Nunain SS, Newell JB, Ruskin JN, William G. Prevalence and prognostic significance of atrial arrhythmias after orthotopic cardiac transplantation. Journal of the American College of Cardiology. 1995;**25**:1673-1680. DOI: https://doi.org/10.1016/0735-1097(95)00047-8

[52] Mathew JP, Parks R, Savino JS, Friedman AS, Koch C, Mangano DT, Browner WS. Atrial fibrillation following coronary artery bypass graft surgery: Predictors, outcomes, and resource utilization. JAMA. 1996;**276**:300-306. DOI: 10.1001/jama.1996.03540040044031

[53] Echahidi N, Pibarot P, O'Hara G, Mathieu P. Mechanisms, prevention, and treatment of atrial fibrillation after cardiac surgery. Journal of the American College of Cardiology. 2008;**51**:793-801. DOI: 10.1016/j.jacc. 2007.10.043

[54] Shingu Y, Kubota S, Wakasa S, Ooka T, Tachibana T, Matsui Y. Postoperative atrial fibrillation: Mechanism, prevention, and future perspective. Surgery Today. 2012;**42**:819-824. DOI: 10.1007/s00595-012-0199-4

[55] Aranki SF, Shaw DP, Adams DH, Rizzo RJ, Couper GS, VanderVliet M, Collins JJ Jr, Cohn LH, Burstin HR. Current trends and impact on hospital resources. Circulation. 1996;**94**:390-397. DOI: https://doi.org/10.1161/01.CIR.94.3.390

[56] Soucier RJ, Mirza S, Abordo MG, Berns E, Dalamagas HC, Hanna A, Silverman DI. Predictors of conversion of atrial fibrillation after cardiac operation in the absence of class I or III antiarrhythmic medications. The Annals of Thoracic Surgery. 2001;**72**:694-697. DOI: http://dx.doi.org/10.1016/S0003-4975(01)02817-X

[57] Lee JK, Klein GJ, Krahn AD, Yee R, Zarnke K, Simpson C, Skanes A, Spindler B. Rate-control versus conversion strategy in postoperative atrial fibrillation: A prospective, randomized pilot study. American Heart Journal. 2000;**140**:871-877. DOI: 10.1067/mhj.2000.111104

[58] Landymore RW, Howell F. Recurrent atrial arrhythmias following treatment for postoperative atrial fibrillation after coronary bypass operations. European Journal of Cardio-Thoracic Surgery. 1991;**5**:436-439. DOI: https://doi.org/10.1016/1010-7940(91)90191-L

[59] Kowey PR, Stebbins D, Igidbashian L, Goldman SM, Sutter FP, Rials SJ, Marinchak RA. Clinical outcome of patients who develop PAF after CABG surgery. Pacing and Clinical Electrophysiology. 2001;**24**:191-193. DOI: 10.1046/j.1460-9592.2001.00191.x

[60] Villareal RP, Hariharan R, Liu BC, Kar B, Lee VV, Elayda M, Lopez JA, Rasekh A, Wilson JM, Massumi A. Postoperative atrial fibrillation and mortality after coronary artery bypass surgery. Journal of the American College of Cardiology. 2004;**43**:742-748. DOI: 10.1016/j.jacc.2003.11.023

[61] Fuller JA, Adams GG, Buxton B. Atrial fibrillation after coronary artery bypass grafting: Is it a disorder of the elderly? The Journal of Thoracic and Cardiovascular Surgery. 1989;**97**:821-825 PMID: 2566713

[62] Lahtinen J, Biancari F, Salmela E, Mosorin M, Satta J, Rainio P, Rimpiläinen J, Lepojärvi M, Juvonen T. Postoperative atrial fibrillation is a major cause of stroke after on-pump coronary artery bypass surgery. The Annals of Thoracic Surgery. 2004;**77**:1241-1244. DOI: 10.1016/j.athoracsur.2003.09.077

[63] Reed GL, III, Singer DE, Picard EH, DeSanctis RW. Stroke following coronary-artery bypass surgery. A case-control estimate of the risk from carotid bruits. The New England Journal of Medicine. 1988;**319**:1246-1250. DOI: 10.1056/NEJM198811103191903

[64] Newman MF, Wolman R, Kanchuger M, Marschall K, Mora-Mangano C, Roach G, Smith LR, Aggarwal A, Nussmeier N, Herskowitz A, Mangano DT. Multicenter preoperative stroke risk index for patients undergoing coronary artery bypass graft surgery. Multicenter study of perioperative ischemia (McSPI) research group. Circulation. 1996;**94**(9 Suppl):II74-II80 PMID: 8901723

[65] Mickleborough LL, Walker PM, Takagi Y, Ohashi M, Ivanov J, Tamariz M. Risk factors for stroke in patients undergoing coronary artery bypass grafting. The Journal of Thoracic and Cardiovascular Surgery. 1996;**112**:1250-1259. DOI: 10.1016/S0022-5223(96)70138-1

[66] Hogue CW Jr, Murphy SF, Schechtman KB, Dávila-Román VG. Risk factors for early or delayed stroke after cardiac surgery. Circulation. 1999;**100**:642-647. DOI: https://doi.org/10.1161/01.CIR.100.6.642

[67] Kim MH, Deeb GM, Morady F, Bruckman D, Hallock LR, Smith KA, Karavite DJ, Bolling SF, Pagani FD, Wahr JA, Sonnad SS, Kazanjian PE, Watts C, Williams M, Eagle KA. Effect of postoperative atrial fibrillation on length of stay after cardiac surgery (the postoperative atrial fibrillation in cardiac surgery study [PACS2]). The American Journal of Cardiology. 2001;**87**:881-885. DOI: http://dx.doi.org/10.1016/S0002-9149(00)01530-7

[68] Lauer MS, Eagle KA, Buckley MJ, DeSanctis RW. Atrial fibrillation following coronary artery bypass surgery. Progress in Cardiovascular Diseases. 1989;**31**:367-378. DOI: http://dx.doi.org/10.1016/0033-0620(89)90031-5

[69] Wyse DG, Waldo AL, DiMarco JP, Domanski MJ, Rosenberg Y, Schron EB, Kellen JC, Greene HL, Mickel MC, Dalquist JE. Atrial fibrillation follow-up investigation of rhythm management (AFFIRM) investigators a comparison of rate control and rhythm control in patients with atrial fibrillation. The New England Journal of Medicine. 2002;**347**:1825-1833. DOI: 10.1056/NEJMoa021328.

[70] Jongnarangsin K, Oral H. Postoperative atrial fibrillation. Cardiology Clinics. 2009;**27**:69-78. DOI: 10.1016/j.ccl.2008.09.011

[71] Mayson SE, Greenspon AJ, Adams S, Decaro MV, Sheth M, Weitz HH, Whellan DJ. The changing face of postoperative atrial fibrillation prevention: A review of current medical therapy. Cardiology in Review. 2007;**15**:231-241. DOI: 10.1097/CRD.0b013e31813e62bb

[72] Al-Khatib SM, Hafley G, Harrington RA, Mack MJ, Ferguson TB, Peterson ED, Califf RM, Kouchoukos NT, Alexander JH. Patterns of management of atrial fibrillation complicating coronary artery bypass grafting: Results from the PRoject of ex-vivo vein graft ENgineering via transfection IV (PREVENT-IV) trial. American Heart Journal. 2009;**158**:792-798. DOI: 10.1016/j.ahj.2009.09.003

[73] Gillinov AM, Bagiella E, Moskowitz AJ, Raiten JM, Groh MA, Bowdish ME, Ailawadi G, Kirkwood KA, Perrault LP, Parides MK, Smith RL II, Kern JA, Dussault G, Hackmann AE, Jeffries NO, Miller MA, Taddei-Peters WC, Rose EA, Weisel RD, Williams DL,

Mangusan RF, Argenziano M, Moquete EG, O'Sullivan KL, Pellerin M, Shah KJ, Gammie JS, Mayer ML, Voisine P, Gelijns AC, O'Gara PT, Mack MJ, CTSN. Rate control versus rhythm control for atrial fibrillation after cardiac surgery. The New England Journal of Medicine. 2016;**374**:1911-1921. DOI: 10.1056/NEJMoa1602002.

[74] January CT, Wann LS, Alpert JS, Calkins H, Cigarroa JE, Cleveland JC Jr, Conti JB, Ellinor PT, Ezekowitz MD, Field ME, Murray KT, Sacco RL, Stevenson WG, Tchou PJ, Tracy CM, Yancy CW; ACC/AHA Task Force Members. 2014 AHA/ACC/HRS guideline for the management of patients with atrial fibrillation: Executive summary: A report of the American College of Cardiology/American Heart Association Task Force on Practice Guidelines and the Heart Rhythm Society. Circulation 2014;**130**:2071-2104. DOI: 10.1161/CIR.0000000000000040

[75] Kirchhof P, Benussi S, Kotecha D, Ahlsson A, Atar D, Casadei B, Castellá M, Diener HC, Heidbuchel H, Hendriks J, Hindricks G, Manolis AS, Oldgren J, Alexandru Popescu B, Schotten U, Van Putte B, Vardas P. 2016 ESC guidelines for the management of atrial fibrillation developed in collaboration with EACTS. European Heart Journal. 2016 Oct 7;**37**(38):2893-2962. DOI: 10.1093/eurheartj/ehw210

[76] Clemo HF, Wood MA, Gilligan DM, Ellenbogen KA. Intravenous amiodarone for acute heart rate control in the critically ill patient with atrial tachyarrhythmias. The American Journal of Cardiology. 1998;**81**:594-598. DOI: http://dx.doi.org/10.1016/S0002-9149(97)00962-4

[77] Daoud EG, Strickberger SA, Man KC, Goyal R, Deeb GM, Bolling SF, Pagani FD, Bitar C, Meissner MD, Morady F. Preoperative amiodarone as prophylaxis against atrial fibrillation after heart surgery. The New England Journal of Medicine. 1997;**337**:1785-1791. DOI: 10.1056/NEJM199712183372501

[78] Dunning J, Treasure T, Versteegh M, Nashef SA, EACTS Audit and Guidelines Committee. Guidelines on the prevention and management of de novo atrial fibrillation after cardiac and thoracic surgery. European Journal of Cardiothoracic Surgery. 2006;**30**:852-872. DOI: 10.1016/j.ejcts.2006.09.003

[79] Heldal M, Atar D. Pharmacological conversion of recent-onset atrial fibrillation: A systematic review. Scandinavian Cardiovascular Journal. Supplement. 2013;**47**:2-10. DOI: 10.3109/14017431.2012.740572

[80] Kowey PR, Dorian P, Mitchell LB, Pratt CM, Roy D, Schwartz PJ, Sadowski J, Sobczyk D, Bochenek A, Toft E, Atrial Arrhythmia Conversion Trial Investigators. Vernakalant hydrochloride for the rapid conversion of atrial fibrillation after cardiac surgery: A randomized, double-blind, placebo-controlled trial. Circulation. Arrhythmia and Electrophysiology. 2009;**2**:652-659. DOI: 10.1161/CIRCEP.109.870204

[81] VanderLugt JT, Mattioni T, Denker S, Torchiana D, Ahern T, Wakefield LK, Perry KT, Kowey PR. Efficacy and safety of ibutilide fumarate for the conversion of atrial arrhythmias after cardiac surgery. Circulation. 1999;**100**:369-375. DOI: https://doi.org/10.1161/01.CIR.100.4.369

[82] Gomes JA, Ip J, Santoni-Rugiu F, Mehta D, Ergin A, Lansman S, Pe E, Newhouse TT, Chao S. Oral d,l sotalol reduces the incidence of post-operative atrial fibrillation in coronary artery

bypass surgery patients: A randomized, double-blind, placebo-controlled study. Journal of the American College of Cardiology. 1999;**34**:334-339. DOI: https://doi.org/10.1016/S0735-1097(99)00213-2

[83] El-Chami MF, Kilgo P, Thourani V, Lattouf OM, Delurgio DB, Guyton RA, Leon AR, Puskas JD. New-onset atrial fibrillation predicts long-term mortality after coronary artery bypass graft. Journal of the American College of Cardiology. 2010;**55**:1370-1376. DOI: 10.1016/j.jacc.2009.10.058

[84] Anderson E, Dyke C, Levy JH. Anticoagulation strategies for the management of postoperative atrial fibrillation. Clinics in Laboratory Medicine. 2014;**34**:537-561. DOI: 10.1016/j.cll.2014.06.012

[85] Arsenault KA, Yusuf AM, Crystal E, Healey JS, Morillo CA, Nair GM, Whitlock RP. Interventions for preventing post-operative atrial fibrillation in patients undergoing heart surgery. Cochrane Database of Systematic Reviews. 2013;**1**:CD003611. DOI: 10.1002/14651858.CD003611.pub3

[86] Khan MF, Wendel CS, Movahed MR. Prevention of post-coronary artery bypass grafting (CABG) atrial fibrillation: Efficacy of prophylactic beta-blockers in the modern era: A meta-analysis of latest randomized controlled trials. Annals of Noninvasive Electrocardiology. 2013;**18**:58-68. DOI: 10.1111/anec.12004

[87] Burgess DC, Kilborn MJ, Keech AC. Interventions for prevention of post-operative atrial fibrillation and its complications after cardiac surgery: A meta-analysis. European Heart Journal. 2006;**27**:2846-2857. DOI: 10.1093/eurheartj/ehl272

[88] Chatterjee S, Sardar P, Mukherjee D, Lichstein E, Aikat S. Timing and route of amiodarone for prevention of postoperative atrial fibrillation after cardiac surgery: A network regression meta-analysis. Pacing and Clinical Electrophysiology. 2013;**36**:1017-1023. DOI: 10.1111/pace.12140

[89] Zhu J, Wang C, Gao D, Zhang C, Zhang Y, Lu Y, Gao Y. Meta-analysis of amiodarone versus beta-blocker as a prophylactic therapy against atrial fibrillation following cardiac surgery. Internal Medicine Journal. 2012;**42**:1078-1087. DOI: 10.1111/j.1445-5994.2012.02844.x

[90] Koniari I, Apostolakis E, Rogkakou C, Baikoussis NG, Dougenis D. Pharmacologic prophylaxis for atrial fibrillation following cardiac surgery: A systematic review. Journal of Cardiothoracic Surgery. 2010;**5**:121. DOI: 10.1186/1749-8090-5-121

[91] Shepherd J, Jones J, Frampton GK, Tanajewski L, Turner D, Price A. Intravenous magnesium sulphate and sotalol for prevention of atrial fibrillation after coronary artery bypass surgery: A systematic review and economic evaluation. Health Technology Assessment. 2008;**12**:iii-iv, ix-95(1-49). DOI: https://dx.doi.org/10.3310/hta12280

[92] Imazio M, Brucato A, Ferrazzi P, Rovere ME, Gandino A, Cemin R, Ferrua S, Belli R, Maestroni S, Simon C, Zingarelli E, Barosi A, Sansone F, Patrini D, Vitali E, Trinchero R, Spodick DH, Adler Y, COPPS Investigators. Colchicine reduces postoperative atrial fibrillation: Results of the colchicine for the prevention of the Postpericardiotomy syndrome (COPPS) atrial fibrillation substudy. Circulation. 2011;**124**:2290-2295. DOI: 10.1161/CIRCULATIONAHA.111.026153

[93] Zheng Z, Jayaram R, Jiang L, Emberson J, Zhao Y, Li Q, Du J, Guarguagli S, Hill M, Chen Z, Collins R, Casadei B. Perioperative Rosuvastatin in cardiac surgery. The New England Journal of Medicine. 2016;**374**:1744-1753. DOI: 10.1056/NEJMoa1507750

[94] Liakopoulos OJ, Kuhn EW, Slottosch I, Wassmer G, Wahlers T. Preoperative statin therapy for patients undergoing cardiac surgery. Cochrane Database of Systematic Reviews. 2012;**4**:Cd008493. DOI: 10.1002/14651858.CD008493.pub2

[95] Fauchier L, Clementy N, Babuty D. Statin therapy and atrial fibrillation: Systematic review and updated meta-analysis of published randomized controlled trials. Current Opinion in Cardiology. 2013;**28**:7-18. DOI: 10.1097/HCO.0b013e32835b0956

[96] Zheng H, Xue S, ZL H, Shan JG, Yang WG. The use of statins to prevent postoperative atrial fibrillation after coronary artery bypass grafting: A meta-analysis of 12 studies. Journal of Cardiovascular Pharmacology. 2014 Sep;**64**(3):285-292. DOI: 10.1097/FJC.0000000000000102

[97] Mathew JP, Fontes ML, Tudor IC, Ramsay J, Duke P, Mazer CD, Barash PG, Hsu PH, Mangano DT, Investigators of the Ischemia Research and Education Foundation, Multicenter Study of Perioperative Ischemia Research Group. A multicenter risk index for atrial fibrillation after cardiac surgery. Journal of the American Medical Association. 2004;**14**(291):1720-1729. DOI: 10.1001/jama.291.14.1720

[98] Cook RC, Yamashita MH, Kearns M, Ramanathan K, Gin K, Humphries KH. Prophylactic magnesium does not prevent atrial fibrillation after cardiac surgery: A meta-analysis. The Annals of Thoracic Surgery. 2013;**95**:533-541. DOI: 10.1016/j.athoracsur.2012.09.008

[99] De Oliveira GS, Jr Knautz JS, Sherwani S, McCarthy RJ. Systemic magnesium to reduce postoperative arrhythmias after coronary artery bypass graft surgery: A meta-analysis of randomized controlled trials. Journal of Cardiothoracic and Vascular Anesthesia. 2012;**26**:643-650. DOI: 10.1053/j.jvca.2012.03.012

[100] Costanzo S, di Niro V, Di Castelnuovo A, Gianfagna F, Donati MB, de Gaetano G, Iacoviello L. Prevention of postoperative atrial fibrillation in open heart surgery patients by preoperative supplementation of n-3 polyunsaturated fatty acids: An updated meta-analysis. The Journal of Thoracic and Cardiovascular Surgery. 2013;**146**:906-911. DOI: 10.1016/j.jtcvs.2013.03.015

[101] Farquharson AL, Metcalf RG, Sanders P, Stuklis R, Edwards JR, Gibson RA, Cleland LG, Sullivan TR, James MJ, Young GD. Effect of dietary fish oil on atrial fibrillation after cardiac surgery. The American Journal of Cardiology. 2011;**108**:851-856. DOI: 10.1016/j.amjcard.2011.04.036

[102] Heidarsdottir R, Arnar DO, Skuladottir GV, Torfason B, Edvardsson V, Gottskalksson G, Palsson R, Indridason OS. Does treatment with n-3 polyunsaturated fatty acids prevent atrial fibrillation after open heart surgery? Europace. 2010;**12**:356-363. DOI: 10.1093/europace/eup429

[103] Mariani J, Doval HC, Nul D, Varini S, Grancelli H, Ferrante D, Tognoni G, Macchia A. N-3 polyunsaturated fatty acids to prevent atrial fibrillation: Updated systematic

review and meta-analysis of randomized controlled trials. Journal of the American Heart Association. 2013;**2**:e005033. DOI: 10.1161/JAHA.112.005033

[104] Rodrigo R, Korantzopoulos P, Cereceda M, Asenjo R, Zamorano J, Villalabeitia E, Baeza C, Aguayo R, Castillo R, Carrasco R, Gormaz JG. A randomized controled trial to prevent post-operative atrial fibrillation by antioxidant reinforcement. Journal of the American College of Cardiology. 2013;**62**:1457-1465. DOI: 10.1016/j.jacc.2013.07.014

[105] Saravanan P, Bridgewater B, West AL, O'Neill SC, Calder PC, Davidson NC. Omega-3 fatty acid supplementation does not reduce risk of atrial fibrillation after coronary artery bypass surgery: A randomized, double-blind, placebo-controlled clinical trial. Circulation. Arrhythmia and Electrophysiology. 2010;**3**:46-53. DOI: 10.1161/CIRCEP.109.899633

[106] Wu JH, Marchioli R, Silletta MG, Macchia A, Song X, Siscovick DS, Harris WS, Masson S, Latini R, Albert C, Brown NJ, Lamarra M, Favaloro RR, Mozaffarian D. Plasma phospholipid omega-3 fatty acids and incidence of postoperative atrial fibrillation in the OPERA trial. Journal of the American Heart Association. 2013;**2**:e000397. DOI: 10.1161/JAHA.113.000397

[107] Xin W, Wei W, Lin Z, Zhang X, Yang H, Zhang T, Li B, Mi S. Fish oil and atrial fibrillation after cardiac surgery: A meta-analysis of randomized controlled trials. PloS One. 2013;**8**:e72913. DOI: 0.1371/journal.pone.0072913

[108] Zhang B, Zhen Y, Tao A, Bao Z, Zhang G. Polyunsaturated fatty acids for the prevention of atrial fibrillation after cardiac surgery: An updated meta-analysis of randomized controlled trials. Journal of Cardiology. 2014;**63**:53-59. DOI: 10.1016/j.jjcc.2013.06.014

[109] Ho KM, Tan JA. Benefits and risks of corticosteroid prophylaxis in adult cardiac surgery a dose-response meta-analysis. Circulation. 2009;**119**:1853-1866. DOI: 10.1161/CIRCULATIONAHA.108.848218

[110] Cappabianca G, Rotunno C, de Luca Tupputi Schinosa L, Ranieri VM, Paparella D. Protective effects of steroids in cardiac surgery: A meta-analysis of randomized double-blind trials. Journal of Cardiothoracic and Vascular Anesthesia. 2011;**25**:156-165. DOI: 10.1053/j.jvca.2010.03.015

[111] Viviano A, Kanagasabay R, Zakkar M. Is perioperative corticosteroid administration associated with a reduced incidence of postoperative atrial fibrillation in adult cardiac surgery? Interactive Cardiovascular and Thoracic Surgery. 2014;**18**:225-229. DOI: https://doi.org/10.1093/icvts/ivt486

[112] Kaleda VI, McCormack DJ, Shipolini AR. Does posterior pericardiotomy reduce the incidence of atrial fibrillation after coronary artery bypass grafting surgery? Interactive Cardiovascular and Thoracic Surgery. 2012;**14**:384-389. DOI: 10.1093/icvts/ivr099

[113] Ozaydin M, Peker O, Erdogan D, Kapan S, Turker Y, Varol E, Ozguner F, Dogan A, Ibrisim E. N-acetylcysteine for the prevention of postoperative atrial fibrillation: A prospective, randomized, placebo-controlled pilot study. European Heart Journal. 2008;**29**:625-631. DOI: 10.1093/eurheartj/ehn011

[114] Cavol Cavolli R, Kaya K, Aslan A, Emiroglu O, Erturk S, Korkmaz O, Oguz M, Tasoz R, Ozyurda U. Does sodium nitroprusside decrease the incidence of atrial fibrillation after myocardial revascularization? A pilot study. Circulation. 2008;**118**:476-481. DOI: 10.1161/CIRCULATIONAHA.107.719377

[115] Fan K, Lee KL, Chiu CS, Lee JW, He GW, Cheung D, Sun MP, Lau CP. Effects of biatrial pacing in prevention of postoperative atrial fibrillation after coronary artery bypass surgery. Circulation. 2000;**102**:755-760. DOI: https://doi.org/10.1161/01.CIR.102.7.755

[116] Daoud EG, Dabir R, Archambeau M, Morady F, Strickberger SA. Randomized, double-blind trial of simultaneous right and left atrial epicardial pacing for prevention of post-open heart surgery atrial fibrillation. Circulation. 2000;**102**:761-765. DOI: https://doi.org/10.1161/01.CIR.102.7.761

[117] Levy T, Fotopoulos G, Walker S, Rex S, Octave M, Paul V, Amrani M. Randomized controlled study investigating the effect of biatrial pacing in prevention of atrial fibrillation after coronary artery bypass grafting. Circulation. 2000;**102**:1382-1387. DOI: https://doi.org/10.1161/01.CIR.102.12.1382

[118] Gerstenfeld EP, Hill MR, French SN, Mehra R, Rofino K, Vander Salm TJ, Mittleman RS. Evaluation of right atrial and biatrial temporary pacing for the prevention of atrial fibrillation after coronary artery bypass surgery. Journal of the American College of Cardiology. 1999;**33**:1981-1988. DOI: https://doi.org/10.1161/01.CIR.102.12.1382

[119] Chung MK, Augostini RS, Asher CR, Pool DP, Grady TA, Zikri M, Buehner SM, Weinstock M, McCarthy PM. Ineffectiveness and potential proarrhythmia of atrial pacing for atrial fibrillation prevention after coronary artery bypass grafting. The Annals of Thoracic Surgery. 2000;**69**:1057-1063. DOI: http://dx.doi.org/10.1016/S0003-4975(99)01338-7

[120] Mori SS, Fujii GG, Ishida HH, Tomari SS, Matsuura AA, Yoshida KK. Atrial flutter after coronary artery bypass grafting: Proposed mechanism as illuminated by independent predictors. Annals of Thoracic and Cardiovascular Surgery. 2003;**9**:50-56 PMID: 12667130

[121] Pap R, Kohári M, Makai A, Bencsik G, Traykov VB, Gallardo R, Klausz G, Zsuzsanna K, Forster T, Sághy L. Surgical technique and the mechanism of atrial tachycardia late after open heart surgery. Journal of Interventional Cardiac Electrophysiology. 2012;**35**:127-135. DOI: 10.1007/s10840-012-9705-2

[122] Hammon JW, Hines MH. Extracorporeal circulation: Perfusion system. In Cohn LH editor. Cardiac Surgery in the Adult. 4th ed. New York: McGraw-Hill; 2008. pp. 350-370. Ch12

[123] Anné W, van Rensburg H, Adams J, Ector H, Van de Werf F, Heidbüchel H. Ablation of post-surgical intra-atrial reentrant tachycardia. Predilection target sites and mapping approach. European Heart Journal. 2002:**23**;1609-1616. PMID: 12323161

[124] Nakagawa H, Shah N, Matsudaira K, Overholt E, Chandrasekaran K, Beckman KJ, Spector P, Calame JD, Rao A, Hasdemir C, Otomo K, Wang Z, Lazzara R, Jackman WM. Characterization of reentrant circuit in macroreentrant right atrial tachycardia after surgical repair of congenital heart disease: Isolated channels between scars allow "focal" ablation. Circulation. 2001 Feb 6;**103**:699-709. DOI: https://doi.org/10.1161/01.CIR.103.5.699

[125] Stewart AM, Greaves K, Bromilow J. Supraventricular tachyarrhythmias and their management in the perioperative period. Continuing Education in Anesthesia, Critical Care and Pain. 2015;**15**:90-97. DOI: https://doi.org/10.1093/bjaceaccp/mku018

[126] Delacrétaz E. Clinical practice. Supraventricular tachycardia. The New England Journal of Medicine. 2006;**354**:1039-1051. DOI: 10.1056/NEJMcp051145

[127] Poldermans D, Bax JJ, Boersma E, De Hert S, Eeckhout E, Fowkes G, Gorenek B, Hennerici MG, Iung B, Kelm M, Kjeldsen KP, Kristensen SD, Lopez-Sendon J, Pelosi P, Philippe F, Pierard L, Ponikowski P, Schmid JP, Sellevold OF, Sicari R, Van den Berghe G, Vermassen F, Hoeks SE, Vanhorebeek I, Vahanian A, Auricchio A, Bax JJ, Ceconi C, Dean V, Filippatos G, Funck-Brentano C, Hobbs R, Kearn P, McDonag T, McGregor K, Popescu BA, Reiner Z, Sechtem U, Sirnes PA, Tendera M, Vardas P, Widimsky P, De Caterina R, Agewall S, Al Attar N, Andreotti F, Anker SD, Baron-Esquivias G, Berkenboom G, Chapoutot L, Cifkova R, Faggiano P, Gibbs S, Hansen HS, Iserin L, Israel CW, Kornowski R, Eizagaechevarria NM, Pepi M, Piepoli M, Priebe HJ, Scherer M, Stepinska J, Taggart D, Tubaro M, Task Force for Preoperative Cardiac Risk Assessment and Perioperative Cardiac Management in Non-cardiac Surgery of European Society of Cardiology (ESC), European Society of Anaesthesiology (ESA). Guidelines for pre-operative cardiac risk assessment and perioperative cardiac Management in non-Cardiac Surgery. The task force for preoperative cardiac risk assessment and perioperative cardiac management in non-cardiac surgery of the European Society of Cardiology (ESC) and endorsed by the European Society of Anaesthesiology (ESA). European Journal of Anaesthesiology. 2010;**27**:92-137. DOI: 10.1097/EJA.0b013e328334c017

[128] Polanczyk CA, Goldman L, Marcantonio ER, Orav EJ, Lee TH. Supraventricular arrhythmia in patients having noncardiac surgery: Clinical correlates and effect on length of stay. Annals of Internal Medicine. 1998;**129**:279-285. DOI: 10.7326/0003-4819-129-4-199808150-00003

[129] Amar D. Perioperative atrial tachyarrhythmias. Anesthesiology. 2002;**97**:1618-1623 PMID: 12459693

[130] Amar D, Roistacher N, Burt M, Reinsel RA, Ginsberg RJ, Wilson RS. Clinical and echocardiographic correlates of symptomatic tachydysrhythmias after noncardiac thoracic surgery. Chest. 1995;**108**:349-354. DOI: https://doi.org/10.1378/chest.108.2.349

[131] Maisel WH, Rawn JD, Stevenson WG. Atrial fibrillation after cardiac surgery. Annals of Internal Medicine. 2001;**18**(135):1061-1073. DOI: 10.7326/0003-4819-135-12-200112180-00010

[132] Roth A, Elkayam I, Shapira I, Sander J, Malov N, Kehati M, Golovner M. Effectiveness of prehospital synchronous direct-current cardioversion for supraventricular tachyarrhythmias causing unstable hemodynamic states. The American Journal of Cardiology. 2003;**91**:489-491. DOI: http://dx.doi.org/10.1016/S0002-9149(02)03257-5

[133] Page RL, Joglar JA, Caldwell MA, Calkins H, Conti JB, Deal BJ, Estes NA 3rd, Field ME, Goldberger ZD, Hammill SC, Indik JH, Lindsay BD, Olshansky B, Russo AM, Shen WK, Tracy CM, Al-Khatib SM. 2015 ACC/AHA/HRS guideline for the Management of

Adult Patients with Supraventricular Tachycardia: A report of the American College of Cardiology/American Heart Association task force on clinical practice guidelines and the Heart Rhythm Society. Journal of the American College of Cardiology. 2016;**67**(13):e27-e115. DOI: 10.1016/j.jacc.2015.08.856

[134] Ascione R, Reeves BC, Santo K, Khan N, Angelini G. Predictors of new malignant ventricular arrhythmias after coronary surgery: A case control study. Journal of the American College of Cardiology. 2004;**43**:1630-1638. DOI: 10.1016/j.jacc.2003.11.056

[135] Huikuri HV, Yli-Mäyry S, Korhonen UR, Airaksinen KE, Ikäheimo MJ, Linnaluoto MK, Takkunen JT. Prevalence and prognostic significance of complex ventricular arrhythmias after coronary arterial bypass graft surgery. International Journal of Cardiology. 1990;**27**:333-339. DOI: 10.1016/0167-5273(90)90290-L

[136] Smith RC, Leung JM, Keith FM, Merrick S, Mangano DT, Study of Perioperative Ischemia (SPI) Research Group. Ventricular dysrhythmias in patients undergoing coronary artery bypass graft surgery: Incidence, characteristics, and prognostic importance. American Heart Journal. 1992;**123**:73-81. DOI: https://doi.org/10.1016/0002-8703(92)90749-L

[137] Pinto RP, Romerill DB, Nasser WK, Schier JJ, Surawicz B. Prognosis of patients with frequent premature ventricular complexes and nonsustained ventricular tachycardia after coronary artery bypass graft surgery. Clinical Cardiology. 1996;**19**:321-324. DOI: 10.1002/clc.4960190408

[138] Topol EJ, Lerman BB, Baughman KL, Platia EV, Griffith LS. De novo refractory ventricular tachyarrhythmias after coronary revascularization. The American Journal of Cardiology. 1986;**57**:57-59. DOI: http://dx.doi.org/10.1016/0002-9149(86)90951-3

[139] King FG, Addetia AM, Peters SD, Peachey GO. Prophylactic lidocaine for postoperative coronary artery bypass patients, a double-blind, randomized trial. Canadian Journal of Anaesthesia. 1990;**37**:363-368. DOI: 10.1007/BF03005592

[140] Chung MK. Cardiac surgery: Postoperative arrhythmias. Critical Care Medicine. 2000;**28**(10):N136-N144 PMID: 11055682

[141] Sapin PM, Woelfel AK, Foster JR. Unexpected ventricular tachyarrhythmias soon after cardiac surgery. The American Journal of Cardiology. 1991;**68**(10):1099-1100. DOI: http://dx.doi.org/10.1016/0002-9149(91)90505-F

[142] Steinberg JS, Gaur A, Sciacca R, Tan E. New-onset sustained ventricular tachycardia after cardiac surgery. Circulation. 1999;**99**:903-908. DOI: https://doi.org/10.1161/01.CIR.99.7.903

[143] Yeung-Lai-Wah JA, Qi A, McNeill E, Abel JG, Tung S, Humphries KH, Kerr CR. New-onset sustained ventricular tachycardia and fibrillation early after cardiac operations. The Annals of Thoracic Surgery. 2004;**77**:2083-2088. DOI: 10.1016/j.athoracsur.2003.12.020

[144] Josephson ME. Recurrent ventricular tachycardia. In: Josephson ME, editor. Clinical Cardiac Electrophysiology: Techniques and Interpretations. 4th ed. Philadelphia: Lippincott Williams &Wilkins; 2008. pp. 446-642

[145] Carmeliet E. Cardiac ionic currents and acute ischemia: From channels to arrhythmias. Physiological Reviews. 1999;**79**:917-1017 PMID: 10390520

[146] Rubart M, Zipes DP. Mechanisms of sudden cardiac death. The Journal of Clinical Investigation. 2005;**115**:2305-2315. DOI: 10.1172/JCI26381

[147] Coronel R, Wilms-Schopman FJ, Dekker LR, Janse MJ. Heterogeneities in [K+]o and TQ potential and the inducibility of ventricular fibrillation during acute regional ischemia in the isolated perfused porcine heart. Circulation. 1995;**92**:120-129. DOI: https://doi.org/10.1161/01.CIR.92.1.120

[148] El-Chami MF, Sawaya FJ, Kilgo P, Stein W 4th, Halkos M, Thourani V, Lattouf OM, Delurgio DB, Guyton RA, Puskas JD, Leon AR.Ventricular arrhythmia after cardiac surgery: Incidence, predictors, and outcomes. Journal of the American College of Cardiology. 2012;**60**:2664-2671. DOI: 10.1016/j.jacc.2012.08.1011

[149] Miller J, Das M. Differential diagnosis for wide QRS complex tachycardia. In: Zipes D, Jalife J, editors. Cardiac Electrophysiology: From Cell to Bedside. 5th ed. Philadelphia: Elsevier International;2010. P.823-831.

[150] Zipes DP, Camm AJ, Borggrefe M, Buxton AE, Chaitman B, Fromer M, Gregoratos G, Klein G, Moss AJ, Myerburg RJ, Priori SG, Quinones MA, Roden DM, Silka MJ, Tracy C, Priori SG, Blanc JJ, Budaj A, Dean V, Deckers JW, Despres C, Dickstein K, Lekakis J, McGregor K, Metra M, Morais J, Osterspey A, Tamargo JL, Zamorano JL, Smith SC Jr, Jacobs AK, Adams CD, Antman EM, Anderson JL, Hunt SA, Halperin JL, Nishimura R, Ornato JP, Page RL, Riegel B; American College of Cardiology; American Heart Association Task Force; European Society of Cardiology Committee for Practice Guidelines; European Heart Rhythm Association; Heart Rhythm Society. ACC/AHA/ESC 2006 guidelines for management of patients with ventricular arrhythmias and the prevention of sudden cardiac death: A report of the American College of Cardiology/American Heart Association task force and the European Society of Cardiology Committee for practice guidelines (writing committee to develop guidelines for management of patients with ventricular arrhythmias and the prevention of sudden cardiac death) developed in collaboration with the European Heart Rhythm Association and the Heart Rhythm Society. Europace. 2006;**8**:746-837. DOI: 10.1093/europace/eul108

[151] Benito B, Josephson ME. Rev Esp Cardiol (Engl Ed). 2012;**65**:939-955. DOI: 10.1016/j.recesp.2012.03.027

[152] Moss AJ, Hall WJ, Cannom DS, Daubert JP, Higgins SL, Klein H, Levine JH, Saksena S, Waldo AL, Wilber D, Brown MW, Heo M. Improved survival with an implanted defibrillator in patients with coronary disease at high risk for ventricular arrhythmia. The New England Journal of Medicine. 1996 Dec;**335**(26, 26):1933-1940. DOI: 10.1056/NEJM199612263352601

[153] Fogel RI, Prystowsky EN. Management of malignant ventricular arrhythmias and cardiac arrest. Critical Care Medicine. 2000;**28**:N165-N169 PMID: 11055686

[154] Rousou JA, Engelman RM, Flack JE 3rd, Deaton DW, Owen SG. Emergency cardiopulmonary bypass in the cardiac surgical unit can be a lifesaving measure in postoperative cardiac arrest. Circulation. 1994;**90**:280-284. PMID: 7955266

[155] Buxton AE, Lee KL, Fisher JD, Josephson ME, Prystowsky EN, Hafley G. A randomized study of the prevention of sudden death in patients with coronary artery disease. The New England Journal of Medicine. 1999;**341**:1882-1890. DOI: 10.1056/NEJM199912163412503

[156] Moss AJ, Zareba W, Hall WJ, Klein H, Wilber DJ, Cannom DS, Daubert JP, Higgins SL, Brown MW, Andrews ML, for the Multicenter Automatic Defibrillator Implantation Trial II Investigators. Prophylactic implantation of a defibrillator in patients with myocardial infarction and reduced ejection fraction. The New England Journal of Medicine. 2002;**346**:877-883. DOI: 10.1056/NEJMoa013474

[157] Bardy GH, Lee KL, Mark DB, Poole JE, Packer DL, Boineau R, Domanski M, Troutman C, Anderson J, Johnson G, McNulty SE, Clapp-Channing N, Davidson-Ray LD, Fraulo ES, Fishbein DP, Luceri RM, Ip JH, Sudden Cardiac Death in Heart Failure Trial (SCD-HeFT) Investigators. Amiodarone or an implantable cardioverter-defibrillator for congestive heart failure. The New England Journal of Medicine. 2005;**352**:225-237. DOI: 10.1056/NEJMoa043399

[158] Goldenberg I, Moss AJ, McNitt S, Zareba W, Hall WJ, Andrews ML, Wilber DJ, Klein HU, Investigators MADIT-II. Time dependence of defibrillator benefit after coronary revascularization in the multicenter automatic defibrillator implantation trial (MADIT)-II. Journal of the American College of Cardiology. 2006;**47**:1811-1817. DOI: 10.1016/j.jacc.2005.12.048

[159] Solomon SD, Zelenkofske S, McMurray JJ, Finn PV, Velazquez E, Ertl G, Harsanyi A, Rouleau JL, Maggioni A, Kober L, White H, Van de Werf F, Pieper K, Califf RM, Pfeffer MA, Valsartan in Acute Myocardial Infarction Trial (VALIANT) Investigators. Sudden death in patients with myocardial infarction and left ventricular dysfunction, heart failure, or both. The New England Journal of Medicine. 2005;**352**:2581-2588. DOI: 10.1056/NEJMoa043938

[160] Zishiri ET, Williams S, Cronin EM, Blackstone EH, Ellis SG, Roselli EE, Smedira NG, Gillinov AM, Glad JA, Tchou PJ, Szymkiewicz SJ, Chung MK. Early risk of mortality after coronary artery revascularization in patients with left ventricular dysfunction and potential role of the wearable cardioverter defibrillator. Circulation. Arrhythmia and Electrophysiology. 2013;**6**:117-128. DOI: 10.1161/CIRCEP.112.973552

[161] Hohnloser SH, Kuck KH, Dorian P, Roberts RS, Hampton JR, Hatala R, Fain E, Gent M, Connolly SJ, DINAMIT Investigators. Prophylactic use of an implantable cardioverter-defibrillator after acute myocardial infarction. The New England Journal of Medicine. 2004;**351**:2481-2488. DOI: 10.1056/NEJMoa041489

[162] Steinbeck G, Andresen D, Seidl K, Brachmann J, Hoffmann E, Wojciechowski D, Kornacewicz-Jach Z, Sredniawa B, Lupkovics G, Hofgärtner F, Lubinski A, Rosenqvist M, Habets A, Wegscheider K, Senges J, Investigators IRIS. Defibrillator implantation early after myocardial infarction. The New England Journal of Medicine. 2009;**361**:1427-1436. DOI: 10.1056/NEJMoa0901889

[163] Morin DP. The Role and Indications of ICD in Patients with Ischemic Cardiomyopathy Undergoing Revascularization [Internet]. 2016. Available from: http://www.acc.org/latest-in-cardiology/articles/2016/03/21/07/42/the-role-and-indications-of-icd-in-patients-with-ischemic-cardiomyopathy-undergoing-revascularization. [Accessed: June 3, 2017]

[164] Bigger JT Jr, for the Coronary Artery Bypass Graft (CABG) Patch Trial Investigators. Prophylactic use of implanted cardiac defibrillators in patients at high risk for ventricular arrhythmias after coronary-artery bypass graft surgery. Coronary artery bypass graft (CABG) patch trial investigators. The New England Journal of Medicine. 1997;**337**:1569-1575. DOI: 10.1056/NEJM199711273372201

[165] Nageh MF, Kim JJ, Chen LH, Yao JF. Implantable defibrillators for secondary prevention of sudden cardiac death in cardiac surgery patients with perioperative ventricular arrhythmias. Journal of the American Heart Association. 2014;**3**:e000686. DOI: 10.1161/JAHA.113.000686

[166] Kusumoto FM, Calkins H, Boehmer J, Buxton AE, Chung MK, Gold MR, Hohnloser SH, Indik J, Lee R, Mehra MR, Menon V, Page RL, Shen WK, Slotwiner DJ, Stevenson LW, Varosy PD, Welikovitch L, Heart Rhythm Society, American College of Cardiology, American Heart Association. HRS/ACC/AHA expert consensus statement on the use of implantable Cardioverter-defibrillator therapy in patients who are not included or not well represented in clinical trials. Journal of the American College of Cardiology. 2014;**64**:1143-1177. DOI: 10.1016/j.jacc.2014.04.008

[167] Moss AJ, Greenberg H, Case RB, Zareba W, Hall WJ, Brown MW, Daubert JP, McNitt S, Andrews ML, Elkin AD, Multicenter Automatic Defibrillator Implantation Trial-II (MADIT-II) Research Group. Long-term clinical course of patients after termination of ventricular tachyarrhythmia by an implanted defibrillator. Circulation. 2004;**110**:3760-3765. DOI: 10.1161/01.CIR.0000150390.04704.B7

[168] Baerman JM, Kirsh MM, de Buitleir M, Hyatt L, Juni JE, Pitt B, Morady F. Natural history and determinants of conduction defects following coronary artery bypass surgery. The Annals of Thoracic Surgery. 1987;**44**:150-153 PMID: 3497615

[169] Goldman BS, Hill TJ, Weisel RD, Scully HE, Mickleborough LL, Pym J, Baird RJ. Permanent pacing after open-heart sugery: Acquired heart disease. Pacing and Clinical Electrophysiology. 1984;**7**:367-371. DOI: 10.1111/j.1540-8159.1984.tb04919.x

[170] Emlein G, Huang SK, Pires LA, Rofino K, Okike ON, Vander Salm TJ. Prolonged bradyarrhythmias after isolated coronary artery bypass graft surgery. American Heart Journal. 1993;**126**:1084-1090. DOI: 10.1016/0002-8703(93)90658-V

[171] Al-Ghamdi B, Mallawi Y, Shafquat A, Ledesma A, AlRuwaili N, Shoukri M, Khan S, Al Saneia A. Predictors of permanent pacemaker implantation after coronary artery bypass grafting and valve surgery in adult patients in current surgical era. Cardiology Research. 2016;**7**:123-129. DOI: http://dx.doi.org/10.14740/cr480w

[172] Miriam S, Leonardo B, Solari Gabriel S. Pacemaker following adult cardiac surgery. In: Min M, editor. Cardiac Pacemakers–Biological Aspects, Clinical Applications and Possible Complications. Croatia: InTech; 2011. pp. 135-160. DOI: 10.5772/23402

[173] Raza SS, Li JM, John R, Chen LY, Tholakanahalli VN, Mbai M, Adabag AS. Long-term mortality and pacing outcomes of patients with permanent pacemaker implantation after cardiac surgery. Pacing and Clinical Electrophysiology. 2011;**34**:331-338. DOI: 10.1111/j.1540-8159.2010.02972.x

[174] Gordon RS, Ivanov J, Cohen G, Ralph-Edwards AL. Permanent cardiac pacing after a cardiac operation: Predictoing the use of permanent pacemakers. The Annals of Thoracic Surgery 1998;**66**:1698-1704. DOI: http://dx.doi.org/10.1016/S0003-4975(98)00889-3

[175] Limongelli G, Ducceschi V, D'Andrea A, Renzulli A, Sarubbi B, De Feo M, Cerasuolo F, Calabrò R, Cotrufo M. Risk factors for pacemaker implantation following aortic valve replacement: A single centre experience. Heart. 2003;**89**:901-904. DOI: http://dx.doi.org/10.1136/heart.89.8.901

[176] Erdogan O, Augostini R, Saliba W, Juratli N, Wilkoff BL. Transiliac permanent pacemaker implantation after extraction of infected pectoral pacemaker systems. The American Journal of Cardiology. 1999;**84**:474-475. DOI: http://dx.doi.org/10.1016/S0002-9149(99)00339-2

[177] Schurr UP, Berli J, Berdajs D, Häusler A, Dzemali O, Emmert M, Seifert B, Genoni M. Incidence and risk factors for pacemaker implantation following aortic valve replacement. Interactive Cardiovascular and Thoracic Surgery. 2010;**11**:556-560. DOI: 10.1510/icvts.2010.249904

[178] Nardi P, Pellegrino A, Scafuri A, Bellos K, De Propris S, Polisca P, Chiariello L. Permanent pacemaker implantation after isolated aortic valve replacement: Incidence, risk factors and surgical technical aspects. Journal of Cardiovascular Medicine (Hagerstown, Md.). 2010;**11**:14-19. DOI: 10.2459/JCM.0b013e32832f9fde

[179] Del Rizzo DF, Nishimura S, Lau C, Sever J, Goldman BS. Cardiac pacing following surgery for acquired heart disease. Journal of Cardiac Surgery. 1996;**11**:332-340. DOI: 10.1111/j.1540-8191.1996.tb00059.x

[180] Sachweh JS, Vazquez-Jimenez JF, Schondube FA, Daebritz SH, Dorge H, Muhler EG, Messmer BJ. Twenty years experience with pediatric pacing: Epicardial and transvenous stimulation. European Journal of Cardio-Thoracic Surgery. 2000;**17**:455-461. DOI: https://doi.org/10.1016/S1010-7940(00)00364-X

[181] Meimoun P, Zeghdi R, D'Attelis N, Berrebi A, Braunberger E, Deloche A, Fabiani JN, Carpentier A. Frequency, predictors, and consequences of atrioventricular block after mitral valve repair. The American Journal of Cardiology. 2002;**89**(9):1062-1066. DOI: http://dx.doi.org/10.1016/S0002-9149(02)02276-2

[182] Heinz G, Kratochwill C, Buxbaum P, Laufer G, Kreiner G, Siostrzonek P, Gasic S, Derfler K, Gössinger H. Immediate normalization of profound sinus node dysfunction by aminophylline after cardiac transplantation. The American Journal of Cardiology. 1993;**71**:346-349. DOI: https://doi.org/10.1016/0002-9149(93)90805-M

[183] Haught WH, Bertolet BD, Conti JB, Curtis AB, Mills RM. Theophylline reverses high-grade atrioventricular block resulting from cardiac transplant rejection. American Heart Journal. 1994;**128**:1255-1257. DOI: http://dx.doi.org/10.1016/0002-8703(94)90764-1

[184] European Society of Cardiology (ESC), European Heart Rhythm Association (EHRA), Brignole M, Auricchio A, Baron-Esquivias G, Bordachar P, Boriani G, Breithardt OA, Cleland J, Deharo JC, Delgado V, Elliott PM, Gorenek B, Israel CW, Leclercq C, Linde C, Mont L, Padeletti L, Sutton R, Vardas PE. 2013 ESC guidelines on cardiac pacing and cardiac resynchronization therapy: The task force on cardiac pacing and resynchronization therapy of the European Society of Cardiology (ESC). Developed in collaboration with the European heart rhythm association (EHRA). Europace. 2013;**15**:1070-1118. DOI: 10.1093/europace/eut206

Chapter 7

Physical Training Programs After Coronary Artery Bypass Grafting

Aikawa Priscila, Nakagawa Naomi Kondo,
Mazzucco Guillermo, Paulitsch Renata Gomes and
Paulitsch Felipe da Silva

Additional information is available at the end of the chapter

http://dx.doi.org/10.5772/intechopen.71978

Abstract

Exercise-based rehabilitation is considered an important adjunct therapy for secondary prevention in patients with coronary artery disease, mainly in populations with coronary artery bypass graft (CABG) and percutaneous coronary intervention. Thus, the increasing number of cardiac surgeries along the years is enlarging the participation of patients in cardiac rehabilitation programs. Encouraging exercise-based cardiac rehabilitation might decreases in-hospital stay, speeds returns to work and reduces costs in public health. Recently, two training modalities of exercise gained much attention in cardiac rehabilitation programs: continuous exercise and high-intensity interval aerobic training (HIIAT). The aim of this chapter is to review the effects of HIIAT in patients that undergone to CABG or other cardiac surgeries regarding clinical and physiological parameters such as death, cardiovascular outcomes, aerobic capacity, anaerobic capacity, quality of life and other parameters, beyond to evaluate the feasibility and safety of HIIAT in this patient's group.

Keywords: coronary artery bypass grafting, high-intensity interval training, exercise intensity, cardiac rehabilitation, physical activity

1. Introduction

At the beginning of the twentieth century, the treatment of heart disease was based on few medicines and unconditional rest over weeks or months. The idea that exercise could overload cardiac pump and increase mortality changed facing the evidence that maintaining physical training and activity under supervision quickly reinsert patients to social-economic life.

This concept could be used for patients in a stable status with acute coronary syndromes, heart failure, post-coronary artery bypass graft (CABG), post- percutaneous coronary intervention (PCI), and most of cardiovascular disease.

Currently, exercise-based rehabilitation is considered an important adjunct therapy for secondary prevention in patients with coronary artery disease mainly in populations undergone CABG and PCI. Thus, physical training was included as Class I recommendation for both healthy subjects and those with coronary artery disease as a central point in cardiac rehabilitation (CR) programs [1–4].

In this chapter, we will discuss exercise physiology, clinical assessments, CR programs and the effects of exercise on cardiac outcomes in patients with coronary artery disease and more specifically patients that undergone CABG.

2. Exercise physiology

Exercise physiology uses some basic principles, and the terms that we will use in the present chapter are described as follows: physical activity as any bodily movement, exercise as physical activity to stress and train, aerobic exercise as exercise that stresses the oxygen transport system, resistance exercise as exercise that stresses musculoskeletal system, and exercise training as exercise performed in a repetitive way to improve cardiovascular (aerobic) or musculoskeletal (resistance) systems. Two main types of exercise have been proposed with beneficial health effects on subjects with CHD: interval aerobic training (IAT) and continuous aerobic training (CAT). IAT uses a balanced or equal time-periods between work and rest. CAT uses a steady-state exercise.

Three variables are important to understand the physiology of exercise: maximal oxygen uptake (VO_2), myocardial oxygen uptake (MO_2), and ventilatory threshold (VT).

VO_2 is the amount of oxygen consumed during exercise, and this variable maintains a closed correlation with the amount of energy used.

Fick describes an equation where cardiac output (Q) = VO_2/difference between arterial and venous oxygen content (ΔA-V O_2). So, VO_2 = ΔA-V O_2 multiplied by Q. Q might be calculated by the product of heart rate (HR) and cardiac stroke volume. Q and ΔA-V O_2 increases during exercise training.

Maximum exercise capacity is measured as maximum VO_2 (VO_{2max}), and it reflects the maximal oxygen transported during exercise before being limited by fatigue or dyspnea. This variable evaluates all together: cardiac, respiratory, muscle-skeletal and vascular systems.

Often diseased patients do not achieve their VO_{2max}, and the term peak VO_2 (VO_{2peak}) should be preferred. VO_{2peak} is the highest level attained by a patient in the absence of fulfilling the criteria for VO_{2max} [5]. The metabolic equivalent (MET) is defined as the oxygen requirement in the resting awake individual, and it is equal to 3.5 ml/Kg/min.

The MO_2 can be estimated multiplying HR by systolic blood pressure, also named double product. MO_2 is not determined by the external work-rate exercise, but rather by the exercise work-rate relative to maximal exercise capacity.

The VT is the divergence of VO_2 and carbon dioxide production (VCO_2) curves, and it is due to production of latic acid. In the beginning of exercise both VO_2 and VCO_2 curves increases in same magnitude. Throughout exercise, the latic acid is buffered by bicarbonate and it increases exhalation of additional CO_2, achieving VT. VT denotes exercise tolerance and represent the maximal constant workrate that can be sustained during submaximal exercise.

3. Cardiac rehabilitation program

World Health Organization defines cardiovascular, pulmonary and metabolic rehabilitation as the integration of interventions called "non-pharmacological actions," to ensure the best physical, psychological and social conditions for the patient with cardiovascular, pulmonary and metabolic diseases.

Based on scientific evidence and proven economic advantages, the ethical medical practice guidelines recommends cardiovascular, pulmonary and metabolic rehabilitation for patients with atherosclerotic coronary disease, heart failure, arterial hypertension, peripheral arterial disease, metabolic diseases (obesity, metabolic syndrome and diabetes mellitus), chronic lung disease, and for subjects with risk factors for cardiovascular diseases such as smoking, dyslipidemia, glucose intolerance, excessive stress, long-term sedentary, and patients with chronic nephropathy. In this context, prescription of training programs is highlighted for the therapeutic benefit of physical exercise which in certain situations should occur under specialized supervision [6].

In the immediate post-operatory period, rehabilitation is based on standard protocols that take more regard the current clinical status and the cardiac pump like left ventricular ejection fraction. Cycle ergometer or treadmill tests are not performed routinely during hospitalization, and the decision to use maximum HR to stop exercise is not suitable. Additionally, most of patients are under beta-blockers and their HR response to exercise will be reduced.

The coordinator of the CR team should focus on several clinical parameters during exercise such as important blood pressure changes—high blood pressure or blood pressure fall during exercise—arrhythmia, syncope or pre-syncope, rales, moderate to severe dyspnea (Borg scale > 14), the onset of angina or claudication. Additionally, upper body motion must be hold by 4 weeks until surgical wound knitting, and 3 or 4 months for pushups and other strenuous exercises.

After the hospital discharge, patients with coronary artery diseases or those that undergone CABG need the referral and the assistant physician consent to perform CR. Before, patients get analysis of their clinical condition and feasibility for performing physical training [6]. Some physicians requiring imaging functional tests like cardiac scintigraphy to assess the baseline perfusion after CABG. The scintigraphy may be performed with a treadmill test or pharmacological stress, like dipyridamole. If the assessment were performed associate to a treadmill test this data can be used as additional information about physiological cardiovascular status, like VO_2, MET, maximal heart rate achieved, chronotropic reserve.

3.1. Phases of CR program

Beyond pharmacological treatment, it is fundamental that patients with heart failure, coronary artery disease or after CABG should be included in an CR program. For the patient's optimal development with improvement in quality of life, it is necessary the participation of a team with different specialties. The CR program aims to improve physiological, clinical and psychological state of the cardiac patient, based on a multidisciplinary intervention of physician, surgeons, physiotherapists, nutritionists, nurses, physiologists, and psychologists.

Secondary prevention and CR are an integral part of the management strategy after revascularization, and it is associated with reductions in morbidity and mortality in a cost-effective way and can further ameliorate symptoms [7, 8].

Traditionally, the CR program can be divided in phases, as follows:

Phase 1: Performed in hospitalized patients. It will introduce the patient to an active and productive life and aims to ensure that the patient will have discharge with the best physical and psychological conditions. Initially, CR was applied for recovery following myocardial infarction or CABG. Currently, it should include patients submitted to PCI by balloon or by stent implantation, heart valve surgeries, congenital heart surgeries, cardiac transplantation, patients with stable angina pectoris and subjects with risk factors for CAD such as subjects with diabetes, hypertension, metabolic syndrome, chronic nephropathy and chronic lung disease. Phase 1 begins after the patient has been considered clinically compensated due to the optimization of the clinical treatment and/or the use of an interventional procedure. In this phase, a combination of low-intensity physical exercise is indicated as well as stress management techniques, and education in relation to risk factors. The duration of this phase has decreased in recent years, due to shorter hospitalizations [6].

Phase 2: This is the first extra-hospital step. It begins immediately after discharge and / or a few days after a cardiovascular event or cardiovascular, pulmonary and metabolic decompensation. Estimated duration: 3–6 months, and in some cases may be more extensive. It can work in a structure that is part of the hospital complex or another environment suitable for physical exercise (sports club, sports gym, gym, etc.). The ideal team should include doctor, physiotherapist, physical education teacher, nurse, nutritionist and psychologist. It must have the basic resources to handle emergencies. It works with sessions supervised by the physiotherapist and/or physical education teacher. The exercise program should be individualized, in terms of intensity, duration, frequency, training modality and progression. There must always be resources for the accurate measurement of heart rate and blood pressure checking, besides the possibility of eventual verification of oxygen saturation, blood glucose determination and electrocardiographic monitoring. Part of this phase is an educational program aimed at lifestyle modification, with emphasis on dietary reeducation and strategies for smoking cessation. The rehabilitation in this phase has as main objective to contribute to the early return of the patient to his social and work activities, in the best possible physical and emotional conditions [6].

Phase 3: Estimated duration of 6–24 months. This is the immediate treatment for the patients discharged from phase 2, but can be started at any stage of the disease evolution. It is not necessary to follow previous phases. Therefore, low-risk patients who did not participate in phase 2 are good candidates. The supervision of exercises should be done by a professional with specialization in physical exercise (physical education teacher and/or physiotherapist), and must be have the coordination of a physician and have the conditions for possible cardiac monitoring and determination of oxygen saturation. It is recommended that other important professionals also integrate the team: nurse, nutritionist and psychologist. The main objective is the improvement of the physical condition and quality of life and other procedures that contribute to the reduction of the risk of clinical complications, such as the strategies for smoking cessation and food reeducation [6].

Phase 4: It is a long-term program, of indefinite duration. Activities are not necessarily supervised and should be appropriate to the availability of time for the maintenance of the physical exercise program and the preferences of patients in relation to recreational sports activities. The material and human resources available should also be considered. At this stage, patients after each medical evaluation, especially when undergoing ergometric tests, should be evaluated and oriented in practice by some supervised exercise sessions. The periodicity to realize the ergometric tests should not exceed 1 year. The main objectives of this phase are to increase and to maintain physical fitness. It is not mandatory that this phase be preceded by phase 3. The rehabilitation team should propose activities that are more appropriate for each one. Patients should be periodically and systematically contacted by the CR team, even by telephone, at least once every 6 months [6].

Within the CR session, each professional can choose to carry out different activities, among which are: aerobic training proper, which can be performed with cycle ergometer, sliding bands, climber or simply with walks guided by trained personnel; resistance exercises, strength exercises, coordination exercises, flexibility exercises and, in phases 3 and 4, specific exercises that have similarity to the work performed by the patient or to the activities performed.

The aerobic training can be performed using two types of exercises:

A. a continuous method (CAT), which is characterized by the application of an uninterrupted load, that means, without pause or periods of rest during the work. This method can be extensive or intensive, finding the difference between both in the intensity of the exercise.

B. an interval aerobic training—IAT method, that contains intervals of rest. When the work is high or moderate intensity, active intervals are used, whereas if the functional capacity of the patient is low, passive recovery intervals are used.

The intensity and duration of aerobic exercises are used to obtain greater benefits for the cardiovascular system and metabolism and have been explored in recent research.

At the beginning of the twenty-first century, research using high-intensity interval aerobic training (HIIAT) was carried out to improve the performance of athletes in competitions.

Examples of protocols of high-intensity interval training (HIIT) applied in studies in trained health volunteers are described as follow:

1. In moderately-trained healthy males. The HIIAT interventions consisted of the following parts: (1) 8 min of a warm-up at a speed of 50% VO_{2max}; (2) interval exercise: total duration of 12 min, work/rest ratio = 1, work intensity 100% VO_{2max}, rest intensity 60% VO_{2max}, work and rest duration of 15 s, 30 s, or 60 s (three different groups); (3) a cool-down: 3 min at 5 km·h^{-1}. All HIIT interventions were identical over the total duration, work/rest ratio, relative work and rest intensity [9].

2. In healthy adults enrolled in non-randomized study. The protocol was low-volume, HIIT consisting of 60 s work and 60 s recovery (60 s/60 s) repeated for 10 repetitions has previously been found to produce beneficial cardiopulmonary, cellular, and metabolic adaptations in healthy and at-risk populations, however using several combinations of work and recovery intensities based in varying percentages of peak power output (PPO) that consisted of the following work/recovery intensities (80% PPO/0% PPO; 80% PPO/50% PPO; 100% PPO/0% PPO and; 100% PPO/50% PPO). In a 100/50 group showed an increasing of PPO and VO_{2max} compared to other groups and, the researchers concluded that use of the 80/0, 80/50, and 100/0 protocols would be appropriate for individuals who are at the low to moderate end of the cardiopulmonary fitness spectrum [10].

3. In healthy young men that performed eight 20 s bouts at 130% of the velocity associated with the VO_{2max} on a treadmill with 10 s of passive rest in HIIT protocol. In this study, the researchers compared to moderate continuous training (MCT), which performed 30 min running on a treadmill at a submaximal velocity equivalent to 90–95% of the heart rate associated with the anaerobic threshold for data related to oxygen consumption and energy expenditure (EE) were measured during the protocols and the excess post-exercise oxygen consumption (EPOC) was calculated for both sessions. The results showed that post-exercise EE and EPOC values were higher after HIIT, suggesting that supramaximal HIIT has a higher impact on EE and EPOC in the early phase of recovery when compared to MCT [11].

The good response to exercise in heath volunteers excited researchers that have been start investigating the benefits of IAT in patients with heart failure during rehabilitation or in patients after CABG. One protocol that showed be effective after CABG consisted of 8 min warm-up, 4 times of 4-min intervals at 90% of maximum heart rate, pauses of 3-min walking at 70% maximum heart rate, and 5 min cool-down after session [12]. This protocol enrolled patients referred to a residential rehabilitation center 4–16 weeks postoperatively, and they excluded heart failure, inability to exercise, or drug abuse. All patients performed a treadmill ergospirometry test before rehabilitation program to evaluation and prescription of exercise intensity and to determine the peak VO_{2peak} pre- and post-training. Ergospirometry is a functional capacity test that noninvasively studies the pathophysiology of the respiratory and cardiovascular systems under conditions of physical stress, objectively evaluating the degree of functional limitation and its mechanism [13]. The ergospirometry have the advantage over conventional treadmill test because it calculates the VT.

Some studies performed the cardiopulmonary test on a treadmill [14, 15], while other studies performed the evaluation on a cycle ergometer [16, 17]. It should be noted that all patients were trained with the same tool with which they were evaluated, both those who performed the test in ergometric bicycle and in the treadmill.

The first IAT study in HF appears to have been in 1972, when patients were asked to cycle on high work load for 60 s with 30 s of rest between intervals. Using intervals, patients could perform the exercises at least twice if they were able to perform on a continuous cycling [18]. Several years ago, most of the scientific evidence demonstrated the benefits of training in patients with HF used continuous low to moderate intensity aerobic exercise. Therefore, few were the professionals who questioned the possibility of using a method that demand greater intensity during aerobic training.

3.2. Benefits of cardiac rehabilitation in cardiac diseases: coronary disease and heart failure

The cardiovascular system response to exercise integrates systemic, cellular, and molecular signaling pathways. The benefits assign to physical training on cardiopulmonary system are improve functional capacity, lessen the intensity of breathing and muscle discomfort, improve quality of life, increase blood muscle flow, increase oxidative and metabolic capacity, attenuate or reverse skeletal muscle atrophy, improve autonomic activation, increase endothelium activation, and improve muscle performance. In this way, it believes that interval exercise training additionally prolongs exercise duration, lowers cardiovascular demand, lowers ventilator requirement, allows higher exercise intensity, and reduces symptoms of dyspnoea and leg discomfort.

A recent meta-analysis [19] from Cochrane Group in CHD concluded that exercise-based CR reduces cardiovascular mortality and provides reduction in hospital admissions and improvements in quality of life regardless of the type of strategy used to treat CHD—medicine, angioplasty, or surgery. Several trials enrolled in this meta-analysis were performed before modern techniques of myocardial revascularization, and it could affect the final results. The GOSPEL study [20] enrolled 3241 patients with recent myocardial infarction and after 3 years of follow-up showed a decreased risk of nonfatal myocardial infarction and combined end-points as cardiovascular death plus nonfatal myocardial infarction and stroke. However, the DANREHAB trial [21] showed no differences between patients with HF, CHD, or high risk heart disease randomized to rehabilitation (n = 380) versus control group (n = 390) after 12 months of follow-up in primary composite outcomes.

The last trial to determine the exercise effect on outcomes in HF patients was the HF-ACTION trial (Heart Failure and A Controlled Trial Investigating Outcomes of Exercise Training) [22, 23]. This trial enrolled 2331 stable systolic HF patients with an EF lower or equal to 35% and randomized them to aerobic training or control group in France, Canada, and United States. Study participants had CHD (51%) and EF (25%). A total of 759 patients (65%) in the exercise group died or were hospitalized compared with 796 patients (68%) in the control group (hazard ratio 0.93 [95% CI: 0.84–1.02]). So, in this sample, the primary and secondary clinical end-points do not show difference between groups. After adjustment for highly prognostic predictors of these end-points, a modest but significant reduction for both, any cause of death or hospitalization and cardiovascular death or HF admission.

In a recent study [24], 261 patients with HF and reduced LVEF (<35%) and NYHA II-III were randomly assigned to HIIT at 90–95% of maximal HR, MCT at 60–70% of HRmax or regular exercise (RRE). In a large clinical trial study, the researchers showed that HIIT was not superior to MCT in changing left ventricular remodeling or aerobic capacity. To access left ventricular remodeling, left ventricular end-diastolic diameter was measured at the tip of the mitral leaflet in two-dimensional parasternal long-axis view by echocardiography and, for aerobic capacity, VO_{2peak} and respiratory quotient were accessed. There was also no difference between HIIT and MCT in VO_{2peak}, but both were superior to RRE. The researchers still reported serious adverse events during the 12 weeks intervention, though there were no statistical significant differences between groups (HIIT 39%, MCT 25%, RRE 34%, $P = 0.16$), numerically was higher in HIIT, followed by RRE and MCT: $n = 82$, 76 e 73, respectively. Therefore, the feasibility of the IAT program remains unresolved in heart failure patients.

Other studies in patients with HF trained in IAT program evaluated variables pre and post-training such as VO_{2max} [7], left ventricular ejection fraction by echocardiographic analysis [7], endothelial function by evaluation of the flow-measured dilation [7], levels of natriuretic peptide in brain plasma, myeloperoxidase, interleukin-6, quality of life by questionnaires SF-36, the Minnesota Living With Heart Failure [8], and the Hare Davis Cardiac Depression Scale [25]. These results were controversial between the group in IAT and CAT programs for some variables.

Although controversies exist for HIIAT in patients with low functional capacity, as in patients with HF, this training method is often the best tool for starting a physical activity program, preventing patients from quickly fatigue and for achieving a better progression during training. Additionally, the HIIAT has been described as feasible to be performed by elderly patients with chronic heart failure and severe alterations in LVEF.

In patients with CAD with preserved or reduced LVEF, HIIAT showed to be superior to moderate MCT to improve VO_{2peak}, which is closely related to long-term survival in cardiac patients [26].

3.3. Benefits of cardiac rehabilitation in patients undergone CABG, focused on interval aerobic training

There are no trials with a sample size that could be considered sufficient to assess the magnitude of effect of exercise training rehabilitation in patients undergone CABG. Regarding IAT versus CET comparisons in such patients, there are only few trials with small sample sizes. Indeed, even with more than 50 years using surgery to treat CHD The scientific evidence of effects of rehabilitation with different protocols on post-CABG management is not extensive [27].

One observational cohort study [28] with 163 survivors' patients after CABG that were followed-up for 5–6 years showed that higher levels of exercise were associated with increased functional status, after adjustment for age, sex, severity of angina, shortness of breath, and fatigue. Interestingly enough, women who did not perform exercise more than 2 times a week had significantly lower physical and social status outcomes than women who did it.

A randomized controlled trial employed to analyze whether a behavioral and educational cardiac rehabilitation program was effective in modifying cardiovascular disease risk factors in 86 patients. The results showed more aerobic capacity assessed by VO_{2max} in the interventional group [29]. Quality of life tended to improve steadily over time in both groups.

In a lack of sufficient trials to evaluate the effect of IAT versus CET as rehabilitation programs on mortality or major cardiovascular events after CABG, few trials with a small sample size used surrogate end-points as hemodynamic and ventilatory parameters to test exercise performance. In this way, VO_{2peak} that strongly predicts mortality and was evaluated in patients submitted to IAT versus continuous moderate training (CMT) after CABG for 4 weeks and 6 months. The VO_{2peak} was measured at the baseline, 4 weeks and after 6 months, presenting similar short-term increases in both IAT and CMT groups. However, there was better long-term effect in IAT group after CABG [12]. Other clinical trial tested IAT versus CET program by 3.5 weeks in a bicycle ergometer protocol. Nine patients in each group performed the exercise 24–26 days after CABG. At the end of protocol, IAT favors increasing physical performance, lower heart rate at rest (−9 bpm versus −4 bpm), lower rate-pressure product at rest, and lower lactate. There were no differences in catecholamines between groups. The authors concluded that IAT is better suited to increase physical performance and is more effective in saving cardiac function compared to CAT [30]. Rate-pressure product were also evaluated by others, and its measures in similar sample of patients with CAD undergone CABG and then trained in either CAT or IAT programs, presented a decreasing in resting and maximal rate-pressure product more significant only in IAT group. The rate-pressure product is an indirect index of myocardial oxygen consumption of patients with CAD [31].

Flow-mediated dilatation reflect the endothelial function and serves as a prognostic marker for cardiovascular events. IAT also enhance endothelial function as observed in studies that evaluated flow-mediated dilation of brachial artery after IAT in post-infarction heart failure [7], but there is a lack of studies with patients after CABG and IAT. In patients with cardiovascular and cerebrovascular disease [32] a systematic review including 20 studies showed that HIIAT was similar to moderate CAT through improvement in endothelial function measured by flow-mediated dilatation, nitric oxide bioavailability and circulating biomarkers.

On the other hand, there is controversy whether physical activity can improve heart function among several cardiac parameters evaluated by echocardiography. One study evaluated patients after CABG [7] and failed to show improvements in systolic annular velocity, mitral annular excursion, late diastolic mitral flow velocity (A wave), early diastolic mitral velocity, late diastolic mitral velocity, deceleration time of the early diastolic mitral velocity ejection fraction, end-diastolic volume, or end-systolic volume after 4 weeks of IAT. The results were similar to baseline, except by peak early diastolic mitral flow velocity (E wave) that it showed significant fall after 4 weeks IAT. However, patients that developed heart failure after infarct, but who did not perform CABG, and undergoing physical training, the IAT showed decline in left ventricle end-diastolic and end-systolic volumes, and left ventricle ejection fraction raised from 28 ± 7.3 to 38 ± 9.8%, with better results to IAT compared to CMT [7].

Regarding changes in blood markers as low-density lipoprotein (LDL)-cholesterol, HDL-cholesterol, triglycerides, glucose, and hemoglobin were not demonstrated or do not have clinical value after IAT in CABG patients [8].

The HIIAT in CABG and PCI patients has been associated with platelet activation (CD62P) and function (platelet aggregation) compared to moderate continuous exercise, showing that the risk of exercise-induced thrombosis is higher during HIIAT than moderate CAT in patients with recent revascularization. Therefore, the acute effect of HIIT on platelet activation and function in patients with recent revascularization is still on debate [33]. In 1990, some studies initiated the research about IAT in patients submitted to CABG [34], but the literature about the theme is still scarce because current researches look for to compare continuous exercise training versus control groups [19]. In this context, it should be emphasized that more clinical trials with patients after CABG are still necessary.

Author details

Aikawa Priscila[1], Nakagawa Naomi Kondo[2*], Mazzucco Guillermo[3], Paulitsch Renata Gomes[4] and Paulitsch Felipe da Silva[5]

*Address all correspondence to: naomikondo@uol.com.br

1 Instituto de Ciências Biológicas da Universidade Federal do Rio Grande, Rio Grande do Sul, Brazil

2 Faculdade de Medicina da Universidade de São Paulo, São Paulo, Brazil

3 Instituto Universitario del Gran Rosario, Rosario, Argentina

4 Universidade Federal do Rio Grande, Rio Grande do Sul, Brazil

5 Faculdade de Medicina da Universidade Federal do Rio Grande, Rio Grande do Sul, Brazil

References

[1] Balady GJ, Ades PA, Bittner VA, Franklin BA, Gordon NF, Thomas RJ, Tomaselli GF, Yancy CW, American Heart Association Science Advisory and Coordinating Committee. Referral, enrollment, and delivery of cardiac rehabilitation/secondary prevention programs at clinical centers and beyond: A presidential advisory from the American Heart Association. Circulation. 2011;**124**(25):2951-2960

[2] Piepoli MF, Hoes AW, Agewall S, Albus C, Brotons C, Catapano AL, Cooney MT, Corrà U, Cosyns B, Deaton C, Graham I, Hall MS, Hobbs FD, Løchen ML, Löllgen H, Marques-Vidal P, Perk J, Prescott E, Redon J, Richter DJ, Sattar N, Smulders Y, Tiberi M, Bart van der Worp H, van Dis I, Verschuren WM. European Guidelines on cardiovascular disease prevention

in clinical practice: The Sixth Joint Task Force of the European Society of Cardiology and Other Societies on Cardiovascular Disease Prevention in Clinical Practice (constituted by representatives of 10 societies and by invited experts) Developed with the special contribution of the European Association for Cardiovascular Prevention & Rehabilitation (EACPR). Atherosclerosis. 2016;**252**:207-274

[3] Eckel RH, Jakicic JM, Ard JD, de Jesus JM, Houston Miller N, Hubbard VS, Lee IM, Lichtenstein AH, Loria CM, Millen BE, Nonas CA, Sacks FM, Smith SC Jr, Svetkey LP, Wadden TA, Yanovski SZ, American College of Cardiology/American Heart Association Task Force on Practice Guidelines. 2013 AHA/ACC guideline on lifestyle management to reduce cardiovascular risk: A report of the American College of Cardiology/American Heart Association Task Force on Practice Guidelines. Journal of the American College of Cardiology. 2014;**63**(25):2960-2984

[4] Wenger NK, Froelicher ES, Smith LK, Ades PA, Berra K, Blumenthal JA, Certo CM, Dattilo AM, Davis D, DeBusk RF, et al. Cardiac rehabilitation as secondary prevention. Agency for Health Care Policy and Research and National Heart, Lung, and Blood Institute. Clinical Practice Guideline. Quick Reference Guide for Clinicians. 1995;**17**:1-23

[5] McArdle A, Vasilaki A, Jackson M. Exercise and skeletal muscle ageing: Cellular and molecular mechanisms. Ageing Research Reviews. 2002;**1**(1):79-93. Review

[6] de Carvalho T et al. Diretriz de reabilitação cardiopulmonar e metabólica: aspectos práticos e responsabilidades. Arquivos Brasileiros de Cardiologia. 2006;**86**(1):74-82

[7] Wisløff U, Støylen A, Loennechen JP, Bruvold M, Rognmo Ø, Haram PM, et al. Superior cardiovascular effect of aerobic interval training versus moderate continuous training in heart failure patients: A randomized study. Circulation. 2007;**24**:3086-3094

[8] Fu TC, Wang CH, Lin PS, Hsu CC, Cherng WJ, Huang SC, et al. Aerobic interval training improves oxygen uptake efficiency by enhancing cerebral and muscular hemodynamics in patients with heart failure. International Journal of Cardiology. 2013;**167**(1):41-50

[9] Cipryan L. IL-6, antioxidant capacity and muscle damage markers following high-intensity interval training protocols. Journal of Human Kinetics. 2017;**15**(56):139-148

[10] Rozenek R, Salassi JW 3rd, Pinto NM, Fleming JD. Acute cardiopulmonary and metabolic responses to high-intensity interval training protocols using 60 s of work and 60 s recovery. Journal of Strength and Conditioning Research. 2016;**30**(11):3014-3023

[11] Schaun GZ, Alberton CL, Ribeiro DO, Pinto SS. Acute effects of high-intensity interval training and moderate-intensity continuous training sessions on cardiorespiratory parameters in healthy young men. European Journal of Applied Physiology. 2017;**117**(7): 1437-1444

[12] Moholdt TT, Amundsen BH, Rustad LA, Wahba A, Løvø KT, Gullikstad LR, Bye A, Skogvoll E, Wisløff U, Slørdahl SA. Aerobic interval training versus continuous moderate exercise after coronary artery bypass surgery: A randomized study of cardiovascular

effects and quality of life. American Heart Journal. 2009;**158**(6):1031-1037. DOI: 10.1016/j.ahj.2009.10.003

[13] Balady GJ, Arena R, Sietsema K, Myers J, Coke L, Fletcher GF, et al. Clinician's Guide to cardiopulmonary exercise testing in adults: A scientific statement from the American Heart Association. Circulation. 2010;**122**:191-225

[14] Smart NA, Steele M. A comparison of 16 weeks of continuous vs intermittent exercise training in chronic heart failure patients. Congestive Heart Failure. 2012;**18**:205-211

[15] Koufaki P, Mercer TH, Keith P, Nolan G, Nolan J, et al. Low-volume high intensity interval training vs continuous aerobic cycling in patients with chronic heart failure: A pragmatic randomised clinical trial of feasibility and effectiveness. Journal of Rehabilitation Medicine. 2014;**46**:348-356

[16] Iellamo F, Manzi V, Caminiti G, Vitale C, Castagna C, Massaro M, et al. Matched dose interval and continuous exercise training induce similar cardiorespiratory and metabolic adaptations in patients with heart failure. International Journal of Cardiology. 2013;**167**(6):2561-2565

[17] Iellamo F, Caminiti G, Sposato B, Vitale C, Massaro M, Rosano G, Volterrani M. Effect of High-Intensity interval training versus moderate continuous training on 24-h blood pressure profile and insulin resistance in patients with chronic heart failure. Internal and Emergency Medicine. 2014;**9**:547-552

[18] Smodlaka VN. Use of the interval work capacity test in the evaluation of severely disabled patients. Journal of Chronic Diseases. 1972;**25**:345-352

[19] Anderson L, Oldridge N, Thompson DR, Zwisler AD, Rees K, Martin N, Taylor RS. Exercise-based cardiac rehabilitation for coronary heart disease: Cochrane systematic review and meta-analysis. Journal of the American College of Cardiology. 2016;5;**67**(1): 1-12

[20] Giannuzzi P, Temporelli PL, Marchioli R, Maggioni AP, Balestroni G, Ceci V, Chieffo C, Gattone M, Griffo R, Schweiger C, Tavazzi L, Urbinati S, Valagussa F, Vanuzzo D, GOSPEL Investigators. Global secondary prevention strategies to limit event recurrence after myocardial infarction: Results of the GOSPEL study, a multicenter, randomized controlled trial from the Italian Cardiac Rehabilitation Network. Archives of Internal Medicine. 2008;10;**168**(20):2194-2204. DOI: 10.1001/archinte.168.20.2194

[21] Zwisler AD, Soja AM, Rasmussen S, Frederiksen M, Abedini S, Appel J, Rasmussen H, Gluud C, Iversen L, Sigurd B, Madsen M, Fischer-Hansen J, DANREHAB Group. Hospital-based comprehensive cardiac rehabilitation versus usual care among patients with congestive heart failure, ischemic heart disease, or high risk of ischemic heart disease: 12-month results of a randomized clinical trial. American Heart Journal. 2008;**155**(6):1106-1113. DOI: 10.1016/j.ahj.2007.12.033. Epub 2008 Mar 14

[22] Flynn KE, Piña IL, Whellan DJ, Lin L, Blumenthal JA, Ellis SJ, Fine LJ, Howlett JG, Keteyian SJ, Kitzman DW, Kraus WE, Miller NH, Schulman KA, Spertus JA, O'Connor CM,

Weinfurt KP, HF-ACTION Investigators. Effects of exercise training on health status in patients with chronic heart failure: HF-ACTION randomized controlled trial. JAMA. 2009;**301**(14):1451-1459. DOI: 10.1001/jama.2009.457. Erratum in: JAMA. 2009;2; **302**(21):2322

[23] Ambrosy AP, Cerbin LP, DeVore AD, Greene SJ, Kraus WE, O'Connor CM, Piña IL, Whellan DJ, Wojdyla D, Wu A, Mentz RJ. Aerobic exercise training and general health status in ambulatory heart failure patients with a reduced ejection fraction-Findings from the Heart Failure and A Controlled Trial Investigating Outcomes of Exercise Training (HF-ACTION) trial. American Heart Journal. 2017;**186**:130-138. DOI: 10.1016/j.ahj.2016.12.017

[24] Ellingsen O, Halle M, Conraads V, Støylen A, Dalen H, Delagardelle C, Larsen AI, Hole T, Mezzani A, Van Craenenbroeck EM, Videm V, Beckers P, Christle JW, Winzer E, Mangner N, Woitek F, Höllriegel R, Pressler A, Monk-Hansen T, Snoer M, Feiereisen P, Valborgland T, Kjekshus J, Hambrecht R, Gielen S, Karlsen T, Prescott E, Linke A, SMARTEX Heart Failure Study (Study of Myocardial Recovery After Exercise Training in Heart Failure) Group. High-intensity interval training in patients with heart failure with reduced ejection fraction. Circulation. 2017;28;**135**(9):839-849

[25] Hare DL, Davis CR. Cardiac Depression Scale: Validation of a new depression scale for cardiac patients. Journal of Psychosomatic Research. 1996;**40**(4):379-386

[26] Pattyn N, Coeckelberghs E, Buys R, Cornelissen VA, Vanhees L. Aerobic interval training vs. moderate continuous training in coronary artery disease patients: A systematic review and meta-analysis. Sports Medicine. 2014;**44**(5):687-700

[27] Coyan GN, Reeder KM, Vacek JL, Coyan GN, Reeder KM, Vacek JL. Diet and exercise interventions following coronary artery bypass graft surgery: A review and call to action. The Physician and Sportsmedicine. 2014;**42**(2):119-129

[28] Treat-Jacobson D, Lindquist RA. Functional recovery and exercise behavior in men and women 5 to 6 years following coronary artery bypass graft (CABG) surgery. Western Journal of Nursing Research. 2004;**26**(5):479-498

[29] Oldenburg B, Martin A, Greenwood J, Bernstein L, Allan R. A controlled trial of a behavioral and educational intervention following coronary artery bypass surgery. Journal of Cardiopulmonary Rehabilitation. 1995;**15**(1):39-46

[30] Meyer K, Lehmann M, Sünder G, Keul J, Weidemann H. Interval versus continuous exercise training after coronary bypass surgery: A comparison of training-induced acute reactions with respect to the effectiveness of the exercise methods. Clinical Cardiology. 1990;**13**(12):851-861

[31] Gaeini AA, Fallahi AA, Kazemi F. Effects of aerobic continuous and interval training on rate-pressure product in patients after CABG surgery. The Journal of Sports Medicine and Physical Fitness. 2015;**55**(1-2):76-83

[32] Kolmos M, Krawcyk RS, Kruuse C. Effect of high-intensity training on endothelial function in patients with cardiovascular and cerebrovascular disease: A systematic review. SAGE Open Medicine. 2016;**4**:2050312116682253

[33] Ahmadizad S, Nouri-Habashi A, Rahmani H, Maleki M, Naderi N, Lotfian S, Salimian M. Platelet activation and function in response to high intensity interval exercise and moderate continuous exercise in CABG and PCI patients. Clinical Hemorheology and Microcirculation. 2016;**64**(4):911-919. DOI: 10.3233/CH-168010

[34] Meyer K, Lehmann M, Sünder G, Keul J, Weidemann H. Acute cardiovascular and metabolic changes in interval and endurance training in selected patients following aortocoronary bypass operation. Zeitschrift für Kardiologie. 1990;**79**(10):689-696

Chapter 8

Medical and Surgical Management and Outcomes for Coronary Artery Disease

Allan Mattia and Frank Manetta

Additional information is available at the end of the chapter

http://dx.doi.org/10.5772/intechopen.71979

Abstract

Coronary artery disease (CAD) is a major cause of death and disability in developed countries. Although coronary artery disease mortality rates worldwide have declined over the past decades, CAD remains responsible for about one third or more of all deaths in individuals over the age of 35 years. Various methods of treatment have been proposed including medical therapy, catheter-based interventions, and lastly, coronary artery bypass grafting. The purpose of this chapter is to outline those treatment regimens and examine the literature detailing their outcomes in hopes of guiding treatment.

Keywords: coronary artery disease, management, outcomes, coronary artery bypass grafting, PCI

1. Introduction: coronary artery disease, an overview and disease burden

Coronary artery disease (CAD) represents a spectrum of clinical syndromes caused by insufficient coronary blood flow to the myocardium. It is almost always due to subintimal atheroma deposition leading to arterial luminal stenosis or occlusion and wall thickening. Coronary atherosclerosis usually involves the proximal portions of larger coronary arteries, especially at or just beyond branching sites. Myocardial ischemia and necrosis occur when coronary blood flow is impaired by atherosclerotic stenosis, resulting in increased oxygen demand. In the setting of symptomatic CAD, compensatory physiologic processes are insufficient to provide adequate myocardial perfusion. The effect is either supply ischemia, responsible for myocardial infarction (MI) and most episodes of unstable angina, or demand ischemia, where coronary blood flow is insufficient during period of increased myocardial demands from exercise, tachycardia, fever, hypertension, or emotional distress [1]. Because the heart has virtually no stores of oxygen and relies entirely on aerobic metabolism, within seconds of coronary occlusion, its high rate of energy expenditures results in a sudden decline of oxygen tension and left ventricular function impairment. The subendocardium is most vulnerable to myocardial ischemia as its collateral flow is lowest; thus, myocardial necrosis progresses toward the epicardium with continued ischemia.

Coronary artery disease is a major cause of death and disability in developed countries. Although coronary artery disease mortality rates worldwide have declined over the past decades, CAD remains responsible for about one third or more of all deaths in individuals over the age of 35 years. In 2017, the Heart Disease and Stroke Statistics update of the American Heart Association reported that 16.5 million persons aged 20 years or older in the United States have coronary artery disease, with a slight male predominance of 55%. In 2013, The Global Burden of Disease estimated that 17.3 million deaths worldwide were related to cardiovascular disease, a 41% increase since 1990 [2–6]. Significant risk factors include but are not limited to age, male sex, hypertension, hyperlipidemia, diabetes mellitus, obesity, tobacco use, family history, and peripheral vascular disease. As one can see, the incidence and prevalence of coronary artery disease are staggering; thus, managing and treating these patients is of utmost concern.

2. Treatment goals of coronary artery disease

The goal of treatment for coronary artery disease is to decrease the frequency and severity of angina symptoms and to increase the duration of one's functional capacity (duration of angina-free exercise). Furthermore, one hopes to prolong life and reduce the incidence of acute coronary syndromes. Such goals are accomplished by increasing myocardial oxygen supply or decreasing myocardial oxygen consumption or both. The reduction in cardiac mortality and incidents of myocardial infarction is achieved by pharmacotherapy and stabilization of atherosclerotic plaques. Comorbid conditions that are treatable could aggravate

Goal	How to Achieve the Goal
Abolish or reduce anginal episodes	Trial of antianginal drugs Coronary revascularization
Increase angina-free walking or exercise	Antianginal drugs Coronary revascularization
Prolong life and reduce acute coronary events (unstable angina, myocardial infarction, coronary death)	Lifestyle modification Modify or correct risk factors Daily aspirin Pharmacotherapy of dyslipidemia Control of hypertension Beta blockers, ACE inhibitors, and CABG surgery in special situations

Figure 1. Management of chronic stable angina.

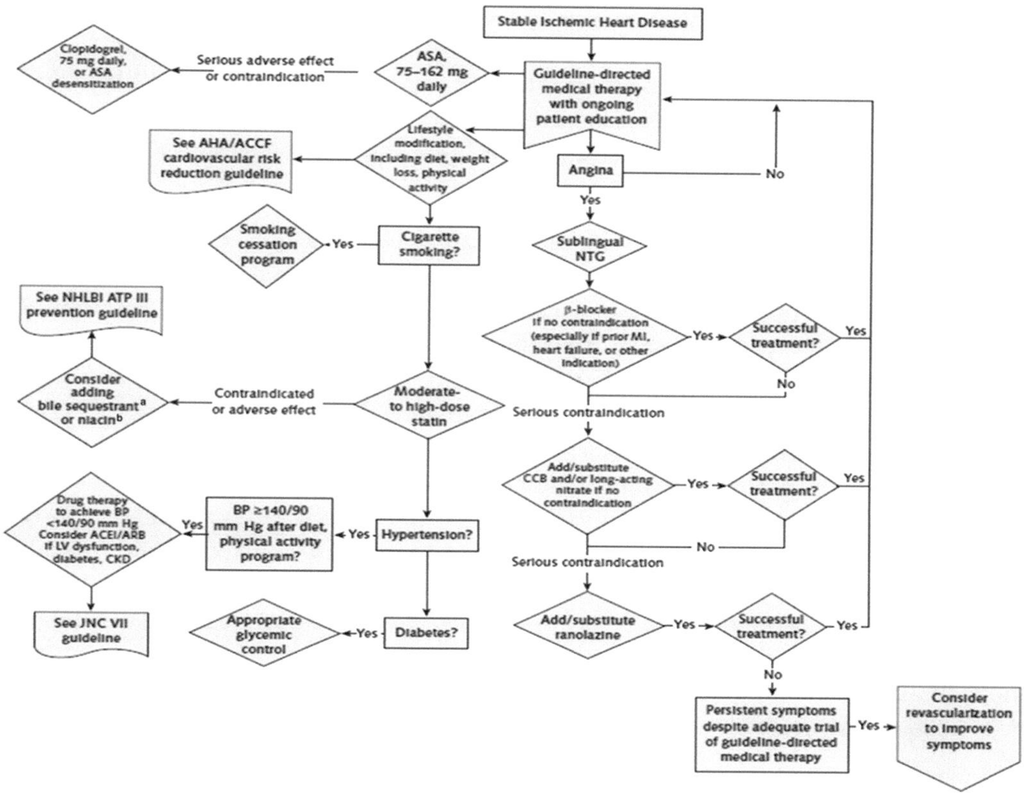

Figure 2. Treatment algorithm for stable ischemic heart disease. *From Ref. [11].

angina, and these conditions must be sought and treated in all patients who have chronic stable angina. There are three options for treatment of stable angina-drug therapy, coronary balloon angioplasty, and coronary artery bypass graft surgery [7–10].

As no two patients are the same, therapy should be individualized and consideration should be given to the risks and benefits of each therapeutic option with regard to symptom relief and longevity. **Figure 1** shows the treatment goals for chronic stable angina and how to achieve them [7–10], and **Figure 2** shows the treatment algorithm for chronic stable angina [11].

3. Medical management of coronary artery disease

From the above treatment algorithm, one can see that there is a large armamentarium at one's disposal for the treatment of coronary artery disease. The uses of these drugs and their mechanisms of action will be outlined below.

Beta blockers have been shown to be very effective in the treatment and management of stable angina. These agents decrease myocardial work and improve exercise tolerance. The primary mechanism of this benefit is through a competitive blockade of β-adrenergic receptors that reduces heart rate and contractility and therefore myocardial O_2 demand. In addition, beta blockers decrease exercise-induced vasoconstriction and blunt the rise in systolic blood pressure during exercise. Beta blockers also increase coronary perfusion by prolonging diastolic perfusion time. Such drugs should be titrated to a heart rate of 50–60 beats per minute at rest and less than 100 beats per minute with exercise.

Calcium channel blockers act mainly by vasodilatation and reduction of peripheral vascular resistance. The nondihydropyridine agents (verapamil and diltiazem), a T-channel blocker (mibefradil), and bepridil inhibit the sinoatrial and atrioventricular nodes and thus also reduce myocardial oxygen demand. The dihydropyridine agents (e.g., nifedipine, amlodipine, felodipine, and nisoldipine) do not affect the sinoatrial or atrioventricular nodes in humans; their mechanism of action is primarily by dilating the coronary arteries and reducing peripheral vascular resistance (and thus reducing myocardial O_2 demand) and by increasing coronary blood flow. Calcium channel blockers block the entry of calcium into the calcium channels in both smooth muscle and myocardium so that less calcium is available to the contractile apparatus. The net result is vasodilatation and a decrease in myocardial contractility. All calcium channel blockers inhibit L-type calcium current in arterial smooth muscle at low concentration and therefore dilate coronary arteries. A major antianginal effect is coronary vessel dilatation and prevention of exercise-induced vessel constriction. Afterload reduction and, in the case of nondihydropyridine channel blockers, the suppressant effects on the sinoatrial node and myocardium also contribute to antianginal efficacy.

Nitrates are coronary vasodilators, and they are anti-ischemic, although the antianginal effects are more far-reaching. Nitrates produce venodilatation, thereby reducing preload, and high doses of nitrates also reduce afterload through arterial vasodilatation. The reduction of preload is secondary to reduced venous return, which in turn reduces ventricular volume and intracavitary pressure and ventricular wall stress. Nitrates can produce dilatation of the site of stenotic coronary lesions and thus increase perfusion to the ischemic myocardium. Nitrates also increase collateral blood flow to ischemic areas. These drugs have not been shown to have an impact on cardiac death from coronary artery disease; however, they have been shown to reduce the rate of angina frequency and increase time to ischemia ECG findings on stress test.

Ranolazine is a selective inhibitor of late sodium influx into myocytes, reducing myocardial contractility. This drug is usually used in combination with beta blockers significantly reducing the frequency of angina and increases exercise duration and time to onset of angina.

Statins are lipid-lowering drugs that work by inhibiting HMG-CoA Reductase. Improvement of myocardial ischemia during ambulatory monitoring has been shown in several studies; however, it is not known whether these agents improve exercise performance [12]. Lipid-lowering agents are recommended for patients with stable angina who have dyslipidemia because these agents have an important influence on prognosis for these patients. High intensive therapy targets an LDL reduction of greater than 50% in high-risk patients and a reduction of 30–50% in those patients who cannot tolerate a high-intensity treatment regimen.

http://dx.doi.org/10.5772/intechopen.71979

ACE inhibitors (captopril, enalapril, and lisinopril) work by inhibiting the angiotensin-converting enzyme. These drugs are a class I recommendation for patients with chronic CAD with LV dysfunction LVEF <40% or diabetes and a class II recommendation for CAD patients without these features [13, 14].

Daily use of aspirin has been shown to reduce the incidence of sudden death and acute myocardial infarction in stable angina. In the Swedish Angina Pectoris Aspirin Trial (SAPAT), daily use of aspirin was associated with a 34% reduction in the incidence of sudden death and acute myocardial infarction, with an absolute reduction of 12 sudden deaths for every 1000 patients treated during the 15-month period [15]. The relative reduction in secondary endpoints (vascular events, vascular death, all-cause mortality, and stroke) ranged from 22 to 32%. There was no difference in major bleeding episodes, including hemorrhagic strokes, between the aspirin and placebo groups. On the basis of these data and available data of the usefulness of aspirin in acute myocardial infarction and unstable angina, it is mandatory that aspirin be used in all patients with stable angina, unless they are unable to tolerate the medication because of either an allergic reaction or intolerable gastrointestinal side effects [8, 16].

Clopidogrel works by selectively inhibiting the binding of adenosine diphosphate (ADP) to its platelet P2Y12 receptor and the subsequent ADP-mediated activation of the glycoprotein GPIIb/IIIa complex, thereby inhibiting platelet aggregation. Patients who are intolerant to aspirin therapy may be treated with clopidogrel. Long-term treatment with a combination of aspirin plus clopidogrel is not superior to aspirin treatment alone and increases the risk of bleeding [17], and it is not recommended for treatment of patients with stable angina. However, combination of aspirin plus clopidogrel for up to 3–12 months after coronary artery stenting reduces adverse clinical outcomes and is indicated in this group of patients.

4. Percutaneous coronary intervention (PCI)

PCI has become one of the most commonly performed medical procedures in the United States, with more than 600,000 procedures performed annually. Over the past decade, the use of drug-eluting stents (DESs) has supplanted the use of older stents, referred to as bare-metal stents (BMSs). Almost all percutaneous coronary interventions (PCIs) performed currently involve stent placement. Thus, although the term percutaneous coronary intervention refers to any therapeutic coronary intervention, it has become essentially synonymous with coronary stent implantation. PCI is performed for coronary revascularization in patients with stable coronary disease as well as, in the appropriate clinical settings, in those with acute coronary syndromes. In **Figures 3** and **4**, one can see a schematic diagram of a PCI [18].

Indications for PCI include:

1. Moderate-to-severe stable angina with evidence of reversible ischemia
2. High-risk unstable angina or non-ST segment elevation myocardial infarction
3. Acute ST segment elevation myocardial infarction

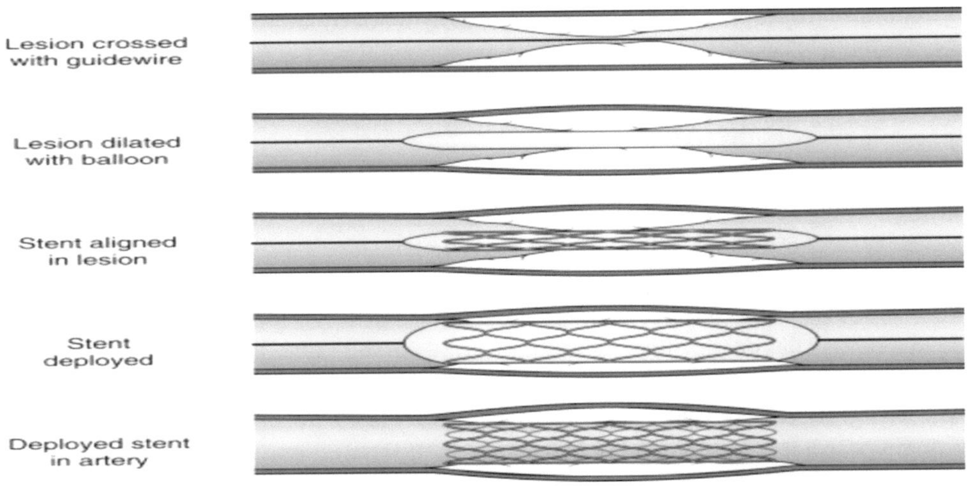

Figure 3. Schematic diagram of a PCI.

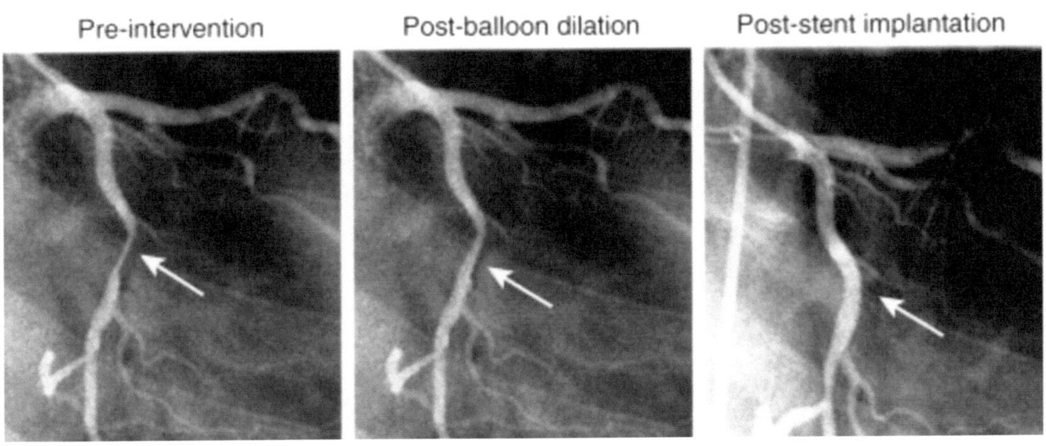

Figure 4. Percutaneous intervention of the circumflex artery seen angiographically [17]. Images from [18].

4. Rescue percutaneous coronary intervention after failed thrombolysis
5. Cardiogenic shock after myocardial infarction
6. Revascularization after successful resuscitation
7. Patients with diabetes mellitus

The only absolute contraindication to PCI is the lack of vascular access or active untreatable severe bleeding, which precludes the use of anticoagulation and antiplatelet agents. Relative contraindications include the following:

- A bleeding diathesis or other conditions that predispose to bleeding during antiplatelet therapy.

http://dx.doi.org/10.5772/intechopen.71979

- Severe renal insufficiency unless the patient is on hemodialysis or has severe electrolyte abnormalities.
- Sepsis.
- Poor patient compliance with medications.
- A terminal condition, such as advanced or metastatic malignancy, that indicates a short life expectancy.
- Other indications for open-heart surgery.
- Anatomic features of poor success.
- Failure of previous PCI or not amenable to PCI based on previous angiograms.
- Severe cognitive dysfunction or advanced physical limitations.

Patients generally should not undergo PCI if the following conditions are present:

- Only a very small area of myocardium is at risk.
- There is no objective evidence of ischemia (unless the patient has clear anginal symptoms and has not had a stress test) with either noninvasive or invasive testing (e.g., fractional flow reserve). One should also beware of false-negative stress tests in patients with left-main CAD.
- There is a low likelihood of technical success.
- The patient has left main or multivessel CAD with a high SYNTAX score and is a candidate for coronary artery bypass grafting (CABG).
- There is insignificant stenosis (less than 50% luminal narrowing).
- The patient has end-stage cirrhosis with portal hypertension resulting in encephalopathy or visceral bleeding.

Following PCI, the patient should be placed on antiplatelet therapy. Patients who are already on aspirin therapy should continue with 81 mg of aspirin daily. Those who are not on aspirin should receive 325 mg of non–enteric-coated aspirin preferably 24 hours prior to PCI, after which aspirin should be continued indefinitely at a dose of 81 mg daily. A loading dose of a P2Y12 inhibitor should be given prior to PCI with stent placement. Following a loading dose of a P2Y12 inhibitor, a maintenance dose is continued. The recommendations for dose and duration are as follows:

- In patients undergoing elective BMS implantation, the duration of P2Y12 inhibitor therapy should be a minimum of 1 month.
- For patient undergoing elective DES implantation (with a second-generation DES) for stable ischemic heart disease, the duration of P2Y12 inhibitor therapy should be at least 6 months.
- For patients undergoing stent BMS or DES implantation in the setting of ACS, clopidogrel 75 mg daily, prasugrel 10 mg daily, or ticagrelor 90 mg twice daily should be continued for at least 12 months. In this setting, ticagrelor and prasugrel are preferred over clopidogrel.

- Shorter duration therapy may be reasonable in patients at high risk for bleeding. Conversely, longer duration therapy may be reasonable in those at higher risk for ischemia but not for bleeding.

5. Coronary artery bypass grafting (CABG)

The decision for surgery is made based on the comprehensive evaluation of the patient. Anatomic considerations that favor recommendation for CABG include presence of significant LM or proximal LAD CAD, multivessel CAD, and presence of lesions not amenable to stenting. The presence of diabetes also favors surgical revascularization over stenting in operable patients. Depressed ejection fraction has been recognized as an additional indication for CABG.

Although the coronary anatomy may be suitable for bypass, each patient's comorbidities should be considered in the overall risk-benefit analysis. Preoperative renal insufficiency, peripheral vascular disease, recent myocardial infarction, or recent stroke, as well as emergency operation and cardiogenic shock, has been identified as factors that increase mortality. The decision to offer CABG or PCI should be determined by a multidisciplinary heart team that evaluates the appropriate therapy on a case-by-case basis.

The current American Heart Association Guidelines for coronary artery bypass grafting can be found in **Figure 5**.

6. A review of the literature: which treatment is best?

Three early prospective randomized trials comparing CABG with medical therapy were conducted in the late 1970s and were reported in the early 1980s. The Veterans' Affairs (VA) cooperative trial, European Coronary Surgery Study (ECSS), and Coronary Artery Surgery Study (CASS) showed long-term superiority of surgery over medical therapy in patients with left main (LM) coronary artery disease, significant coronary artery disease involving the LAD artery, and multivessel disease.

The first study was reported in 1982 in the European Coronary Surgery Study [19]. This study randomized 768 men to medical or surgical treatment. In follow-up extending to 8 years, survival was significantly improved by surgery in patients with significant three-vessel disease and in patients with significant stenosis in the proximal LAD coronary artery who had two- or three-vessel disease. Compared with medically treated patients, late mortality was reduced by 53% at 5 years in surgically treated patients, and among those with three-vessel disease, the 5-year mortality rate was lowered by 66%. In the subgroup of patients with significant narrowing of the proximal LAD coronary artery, the 5-year mortality rate was lowered 60% by surgery.

The second study reporting the efficacy of coronary revascularization was the 1984 Veterans Administration study [20]. This study evaluated the long-term survival after CABG in 686 patients with stable angina, and patients were observed for an average of 11.2 years. The 7-year survival curves for the total population of patients showed a statistically significant survival benefit of 77% with surgical therapy compared with 70% survival with medical

http://dx.doi.org/10.5772/intechopen.71979

AHA/ACC Guidelines for CABG

Asymptomatic/Mild Angina

Class I

1. Left main stenosis
2. Left main equivalent (proximal LAD and proximal circumflex)
3. Three-vessel disease

Class IIa

1. Proximal LAD stenosis and one- or two-vessel disease

Class IIb

1. One- or two-vessel disease not involving proximal LAD

If a large territory at risk on noninvasive studies or LVEF<50%, IIa and IIb become class I indications

Stable Angina

Class I

1. Left main stenosis
2. Left main equivalent (proximal LAD and proximal circumflex)
3. Three-vessel disease
4. Two-vessel disease with proximal LAD stenosis and EF <50% or demonstrable ischemia
5. One- or two-vessel disease without proximal LAD stenosis but with a large territory at risk and high-risk criteria on noninvasive testing
6. Disabling angina refractory to medical therapy

Class IIa

1. Proximal LAD stenosis with one-vessel disease
2. One- or two-vessel disease without proximal LAD stenosis, but with a moderate territory at risk and demonstrable ischemia

Unstable Angina/Non-ST-Segment Elevation MI (NSTEMI)

Class I

1. Left main
2. Left main equivalent
3. Ongoing ischemia not responsive to maximal nonsurgical therapy

Class IIa

1. Proximal LAD stenosis with one- or two-vessel disease

Class IIb

1. One- or two-vessel disease without proximal LAD stenosis when PCI not possible (becomes class I if high-risk criteria on noninvasive testing)

ST-Segment Elevation (Q wave) MI

Class I

1. Failed PCI with persistent pain or shock and anatomically feasible
2. Persistent or recurrent ischemia refractory to medical treatment with acceptable anatomy who have a significant territory at risk and not a candidate for PCI
3. Requires surgical repair of post-infarct ventricular septal rupture or mitral valve insufficiency
4. Cardiogenic shock in patients <75 years of age who have ST elevation, LBBB, or a posterior MI within 18 hours of onset
5. Life-threatening ventricular arrhythmias in the presence of ≥50% left main stenosis or three-vessel disease

Class IIa

1. Primary reperfusion in patients who have failed fibrinolytics or PCI and are in the early stages (6–12 h) of an evolving STEMI
2. Mortality with CABG is elevated the first 3–7 days after STEMI/NSTEMI. After 7 days, criteria for revascularization in previous sections apply.

Poor LV Function

Class I

1. Left main stenosis
2. Left main equivalent
3. Proximal LAD stenosis and two- to three-vessel disease

Class IIa

1. Significant viable territory and noncontractile myocardium

Life-Threatening Ventricular Arrhythmias

Class I

1. Left main disease
2. Three-vessel disease

Class IIa

1. Bypassable one- or two-vessel disease
2. Proximal LAD disease and one- or two-vessel disease.

These become class I indications if arrhythmia is resuscitated cardiac death or sustained ventricular tachycardia.

Failed PCI

Class I

1. Ongoing ischemia with significant territory at risk
2. Shock

Class IIa

1. Foreign body in critical position
2. Shock with coagulopathy and no previous sternotomy

Class IIb

1. Shock with coagulopathy and previous sternotomy

Previous CABG

Class I

1. Disabling angina refractory to medical therapy
2. Nonpatent previous bypass grafts, but with class I indications for native CAD

Class IIa

1. Large territory at risk
2. Vein grafts supplying LAD or large territory are >50% stenosed

Figure 5. AHA/ACC guidelines for CABG.

treatment. This benefit diminished by 11 years of observation, but a survival advantage persisted 11 years in surgical patients with three-vessel disease and impaired left ventricular function and in those at high clinical risk defined by preoperative ST-segment depression, history of myocardial infarction, or hypertension (**Figure 6**).

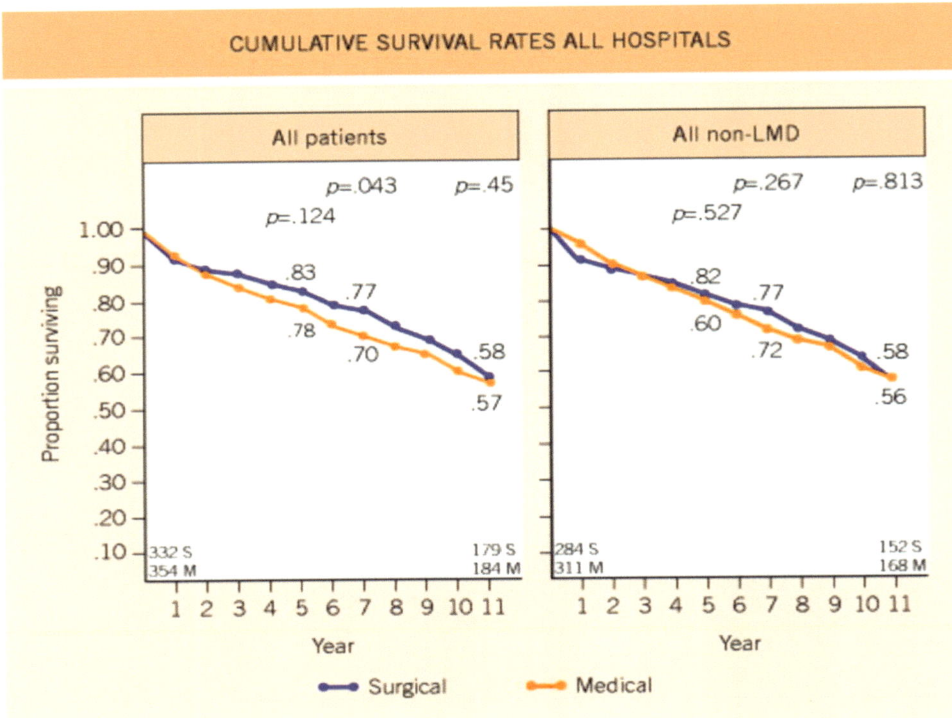

Figure 6. VA study results. Eleven-year cumulative survival for all patients according to treatment assignment. Survival curve for randomized medical (M) and surgical (S) groups in all patients and all patients without left main disease (non-LMD). From Veterans Administration Coronary Artery Bypass Surgery Cooperative Study Group [20].

Finally, the Coronary Artery Surgery Study (CASS) [21] reported survival data of 780 patients with stable angina and ejection fractions greater than 35% who were assigned to receive medical or surgical therapy. At 8 years of follow-up, 87% of surgically treated patients were alive compared with 84% of those receiving medical therapy. Although not statistically significant, the trend favored surgical therapy. Of note, the subgroup with three-vessel disease and a reduced ejection fraction of less than 50% but greater than 35% had a significant survival benefit in the surgical group at 7 years of 88% compared with 65% in the medical therapy group (**Figure 7**).

While the above studies showed the impact coronary revascularization has on patient long-term outcomes compared to medical therapy alone, there remained much debate in regard to efficacy and patient survival when comparing coronary artery bypass grafting and percutaneous coronary interventions. Perhaps, the single most important trial comparing the two interventions was the SYNTAX trial. This trial involved 85 treatment centers and 1800 patients with multivessel or left main coronary artery disease. These showed worse outcomes in the PCI group as compared to the CABG group, with increased composite major adverse cardiac and cerebrovascular events (MACCE: death, stroke, MI, or repeat revascularization). Although there was no significant difference in all-cause mortality and stroke at 5 years, MI and repeat revascularization were both increased in the PCI group. Of note, in patients with three-vessel coronary artery disease (CAD), CABG in comparison with PCI was associated with a significantly reduced rate of MI-related death, which was the leading cause of death

http://dx.doi.org/10.5772/intechopen.71979

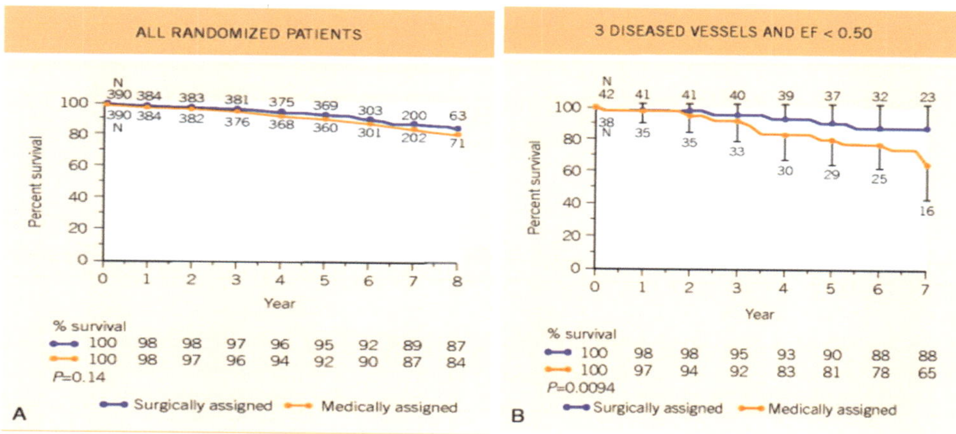

Figure 7. CASS results. Cumulative survival for patients participating in the CASS randomized trial. (A) Survival curve for all patients assigned to medical or surgical therapy and (B) survival curve for patients with three diseased vessels and ejection fractions (EF) less than 0.50 assigned to medical or surgical therapy. From Killip et al. [21].

after PCI. The study concluded that patients with more complex disease (3VD with intermediate-high SYNTAX scores and LM with high SYNTAX score) have an increased risk of a MACCE event with PCI, and CABG is the preferred treatment option.

The syntax score is a scoring system developed by the SYNTAX trial investigators to quantify the extent and complexity of CAD based on findings at cardiac catheterization. Scores are divided into terciles: low (0–22), intermediate (23–32), and high (≥33), with higher scores representing more extensive and complex CAD. The SYNTAX score was found to correlate with PCI risk and outcome but not with CABG risk and outcome. Patients with higher SYNTAX scores generally benefited from a revascularization strategy of CABG in preference to PCI. This is reflected in current guidelines, which state that it is reasonable to choose CABG over PCI as a revascularization strategy in patients with complex three-vessel disease and high SYNTAX score.

It must be noted that for patients with complicated coronary artery disease, coronary artery bypass surgery has been shown to be superior to that of PCI. From the studies above, it can be noted that this difference can be seen after a 5 year follow up period. Thus, for patients with triple vessel disease, diabetes and reduced ejection fraction, coronary artery bypass surgery should be the standard of care.

Author details

Allan Mattia and Frank Manetta*

*Address all correspondence to: fmanetta@northwell.edu

Department of Cardiovascular and Thoracic Surgery, Hofstra Northwell School of Medicine, Manhasset, NY, USA

References

[1] Ganz P, Ganz W. Coronary blood flow and myocardial ischemia. In: Braunwald E, Zipes DP, Libby P, editors. Heart Disease. Philadelphia: W.B. Saunders Company; 2001. pp. 1087-1113

[2] Rosamond W, Flegal K, Furie K, et al. Heart disease and stroke statistics—2008 update: A report from the American Heart Association statistics committee and stroke statistics subcommittee. Circulation. 2008;**117**:e25

[3] Nichols M, Townsend N, Scarborough P, Rayner M. Cardiovascular disease in Europe 2014: Epidemiological update. European Heart Journal. 2014;**35**:2950

[4] Benjamin EJ, Blaha MJ, Chiuve SE, et al. Heart disease and stroke Statistics-2017 update: A report from the American Heart Association. Circulation. 2017;**135**:e146

[5] Lloyd-Jones DM, Larson MG, Beiser A, Levy D. Lifetime risk of developing coronary heart disease. Lancet. 1999;**353**:89

[6] GBD 2013 Mortality and Causes of Death Collaborators. Global, regional, and national age-sex specific all-cause and cause-specific mortality for 240 causes of death, 1990-2013: A systematic analysis for the global burden of disease study 2013. Lancet. 2015;**385**:117

[7] Thadani U. Current medical management of chronic stable angina. Journal of Cardiovascular Pharmacology and Therapeutics. 2004;**9**:S11-S29

[8] Asirvatham S, Sebastian C, Thadani U. Choosing the most appropriate treatment for stable angina: Safety considerations. Drug Safety. 1998;**19**:23-44

[9] Thadani U. Management of stable angina pectoris. Current Opinion in Cardiology. 1999; **14**:349-358

[10] Thadani U. Management of patients with chronic stable angina at low risk for serious cardiac events. The American Journal of Cardiology. 1997;**79**:24-30

[11] Fihn SD, Gardin JM, Abrams J, et al. ACCF/AHA/ACP/AATS/PCNA/SCAI/STS guideline for the diagnosis and management of patients with stable ischemic heart disease: A report of the American College of Cardiology Foundation/American Heart Association Task Force on Practice Guidelines, and the American College of Physicians, American Association for Thoracic Surgery, Preventive Cardiovascular Nurses Association, Society for Cardiovascular Angiography and Interventions, and Society of Thoracic Surgeons. Journal of the American College of Cardiology. 2012;**60**:e44-e164

[12] Tzivoni D, Klein J. Improvement of myocardial ischaemia by lipid lowering drugs. European Heart Journal. 1998;**19**:230-234

[13] Yusuf S, Pitt B, Davis CE, et al. Effect of enalapril on survival in patients with reduced left ventricular ejection fraction and congestive heart failure. The New England Journal of Medicine. 1991;**325**:293-302

[14] Pfeffer MA, Braunwald E, Moye LA, et al. Effect of captopril on mortality and morbidity in patients with left ventricular dysfunction after myocardial infarction. The New England Journal of Medicine. 1992;**527**:669-677

[15] Juul-Moller S, Edvardson N, Jahnmatz B, et al. Double blind trial of aspirin in primary prevention of myocardial infarction in patients with stable chronic angina pectoris. Lancet. 1992;**340**:1421-1425

[16] Food and Drug Administration. Acetylsalicylic acid and the heart. JAMA. 1993;**270**:2669

[17] Bhatt DL, Fox KA, Hacke W, et al. Clopidogrel and aspirin versus aspirin alone for the prevention of atherothrombotic events. The New England Journal of Medicine. 2006; **354**:1706-1717

[18] Levine GN. Color Atlas of Cardiovascular Disease. New Delhi, India: Jaypee Brothers Medical Publishers; 2014

[19] European Coronary Surgery Study Group. Long-term results of prospective randomized study of coronary artery bypass surgery in stable angina pectoris. European Coronary Surgery Study Group. Lancet. 1982;**2**:1173-1180

[20] The Veterans Administration Coronary Artery Bypass Surgery Cooperative Study Group. Eleven-year survival in the Veterans Administration randomized trial of coronary bypass surgery for stable angina. The New England Journal of Medicine. 1984;**311**: 1333-1339

[21] Killip T, Passamani E, Davis K. Coronary artery surgery study (CASS): A randomized trial of coronary bypass surgery. Circulation. 1985;**72**:V102-V109